W9-CDV-386

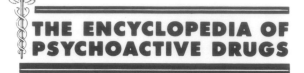

THE ENCYCLOPEDIA OF PSYCHOACTIVE DRUGS

SERIES 1

SERIES 2

CAFFEINE

EDITOR, WRITER
OF UPDATED MATERIAL

Ann Keene

GENERAL EDITOR
OF UPDATING PROJECT

Professor Paul R. Sanberg, Ph.D.

Department of Psychiatry, Neurosurgery,
Physiology, and Biophysics
University of Cincinnati College of Medicine; and
Director of Neuroscience, Cellular Transplants, Inc.

GENERAL EDITOR

Professor Solomon H. Snyder, M.D.

Distinguished Service Professor of
Neuroscience, Pharmacology, and Psychiatry at
The Johns Hopkins University School of Medicine

ASSOCIATE EDITOR

Professor Barry L. Jacobs, Ph.D.

Program in Neuroscience, Department of Psychology,
Princeton University

SENIOR EDITORIAL CONSULTANT

Jerome H. Jaffe, M.D.

Director of The Addiction Research Center,
National Institute on Drug Abuse

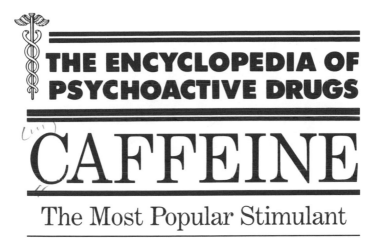

THE ENCYCLOPEDIA OF PSYCHOACTIVE DRUGS

CAFFEINE

The Most Popular Stimulant

RICHARD M. GILBERT, Ph.D.

Addition Research Foundation of Ontario

0 64002

WITHDRAWN

RC
567
.5
.G54
1992

CHELSEA HOUSE PUBLISHERS
NEW YORK   PHILADELPHIA

On the Cover Detail from *Nighthawks,* by Edward Hopper, 1942, oil on canvas, 33 3/16" × 60 1/8", Friends of American Art Collection (Goodman Fund). © The Art Institute of Chicago. All rights reserved.

Chelsea House Publishers

EDITOR-IN-CHIEF: Remmel Nunn
MANAGING EDITOR: Karyn Gullen Browne
PICTURE EDITOR: Adrian G. Allen
ART DIRECTOR: Maria Epes
MANUFACTURING MANAGER: Gerald Levine
SYSTEMS MANAGER: Lindsey Ottman
PRODUCTION MANAGER: Joseph Romano

THE ENCYCLOPEDIA OF PSYCHOACTIVE DRUGS
EDITOR OF UPDATED MATERIAL: Ann Keene

STAFF FOR CAFFEINE: THE MOST POPULAR STIMULANT
PRODUCTION EDITOR: Marie Claire Cebrián
LAYOUT: Bernard Schleifer
APPENDIXES AND TABLES: Gary Tong
PICTURE RESEARCH: Ian Ensign, Jonathan Shapiro

UPDATED 1992
3 5 7 9 8 6 4 2

Copyright © 1986 by Chelsea House Publishers, a division of Main Line Book Co. Updated 1992. All rights reserved.
Printed and bound in the United States of America.

Library of Congress Cataloging-in-Publication Data
Gilbert, Richard M.
    Caffeine, the most popular stimulant.
    (The Encyclopedia of psychoactive drugs)
    Bibliography: p.
    Includes index.
    Summary: Examines the nature and effects, both harmful and beneficial, of the use and abuse of this popular stimulant.
    1. Caffeine habit. 2. Caffeine—Physiological effect. [1. Caffeine. 2. Drugs. 3. Drug abuse]
I. Title. II. Series.
RC567.5.G54   1986   615'.785   82-25970
ISBN 0-87754-756-4
    0-7910-0757-X (pbk.)

Photos courtesy of AP/Wide World Photos, The Bettmann Archive, Dover Publishers, Weatherhill Publishers

CONTENTS

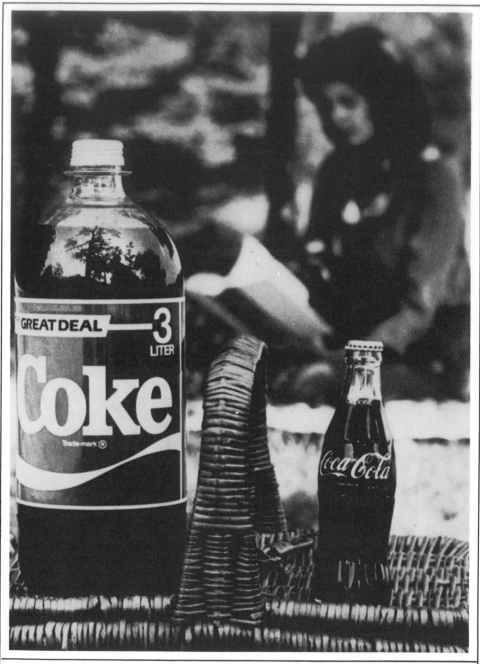

Coca-Cola Classic is the number-one soft drink in the United States, followed in popularity by three other colas: Pepsi, Diet Coke, and Diet Pepsi. A 12-ounce can of cola contains between 38 and 46 mg of caffeine. Caffeine-free cola drinks have been on the market since the mid-1980s, but are far less popular than caffeine-containing brands.

FOREWORD

Since the 1960s, the abuse of psychoactive substances—drugs that alter mood and behavior—has grown alarmingly. Many experts in the fields of medicine, public health, law enforcement, and crime prevention are calling the situation an epidemic. Some legal psychoactive substances—alcohol, caffeine, and nicotine, for example—have been in use since colonial times; illegal ones such as heroin and marijuana have been used to a varying extent by certain segments of the population for decades. But only in the late 20th century has there been widespread reliance on such a variety of mind-altering substances—by youth as well as by adults.

Day after day, newspapers, magazines, and television and radio programs bring us the grim consequences of this dependence. Addiction threatens not only personal health but the stability of our communities and currently costs society an estimated $180 billion annually in the United States alone. Drug-related violent crime and death are increasingly becoming a way of life in many of our cities, towns, and rural areas alike.

Why do people use drugs of any kind? There is one simple answer: to "feel better," physically or mentally. The antibiotics your doctor prescribes for an ear infection destroy the bacteria and make the pain go away. Aspirin can make us more comfortable by reducing fever, banishing a headache, or relieving joint pain from arthritis. Cigarettes put smokers at ease in social situations; a beer or a cocktail helps a worker relax after a hard day on the job. Caffeine, the most widely used drug in America, wakes us up in the morning and over-comes fatigue when we have exams to study for or a long drive to make. Prescription drugs, over-the-counter remedies, tobacco products, alcoholic beverages, caffeine products—all of these are legally available substances that have the capacity to change the way we feel.

But the drugs causing the most concern today are not found in a package of NoDoz or in an aspirin bottle. The drugs that government and private agencies are spending billions of dollars to overcome in the name of crime prevention, law enforcement, rehabilitation, and education have names like crack, angel dust, pot, horse, and speed. Cocaine, PCP, marijuana, heroin, and amphetamines can be very dangerous indeed, to both users and those with whom they live, go to school, and work. But other mood- and mind-altering substances are having a devastating impact, too—especially on youth.

Consider alcohol: The minimum legal drinking age in all 50 states is now 21, but adolescent consumption remains high, even as a decline in other forms of drug use is reported. A recent survey of high school seniors reveals that on any given weekend one in three seniors will be drunk; more than half of all high school seniors report that they have driven while they were drunk. The average age at which a child has his or her first drink is now 12, and more than 1 in 3 eighth-graders report having been drunk at least once.

Or consider nicotine, the psychoactive and addictive in-gredient of tobacco: While smoking has declined in the pop-ulation as a whole, the number of adolescent girls who smoke has been steadily increasing. Because certain health hazards of smoking have been conclusively demonstrated—its rela-tionship to heart disease, lung cancer, and respiratory disease; its link to premature birth and low birth weight of babies whose mothers smoked during pregnancy—the long-term ef-fects of such a trend are a cause for concern.

Studies have shown that almost all drug abuse begins in the preteen and teenage years. It is not difficult to understand why: Adolescence is a time of tremendous change and tur-moil, when teenagers face the tasks of discovering their iden-tity, clarifying their sexual roles, asserting their independence as they learn to cope with authority, and searching for goals. The pressures—from friends, parents, teachers, coaches, and one's own self—are great, and the temptation to want to "feel better" by taking drugs is powerful.

Psychoactive drugs are everywhere in our society, and their use and misuse show no sign of waning. The lack of success in the so-called war on drugs, begun in earnest in the 1980s, has shown us that we cannot "drug proof" our homes, schools, workplaces, and communities. What we can do, however, is make available the latest information on these substances and their effects and ask that those reading it consider the information carefully.

The newly updated ENCYCLOPEDIA OF PSYCHOACTIVE DRUGS, specifically written for young people, provides up-to-date information on a variety of substances that are widely abused in today's society. Each volume is devoted to a specific substance or pattern of abuse and is designed to answer the questions that young readers are likely to ask about drugs. An individualized glossary in each volume defines key words and terms, and newly enlarged and updated appendixes include recent statistical data as well as a special section on AIDS and its relation to drug abuse. The editors of the EN-CYCLOPEDIA OF PSYCHOACTIVE DRUGS hope this series will help today's adolescents make intelligent choices as they prepare for maturity in the 21st century.

Ann Keene, Editor

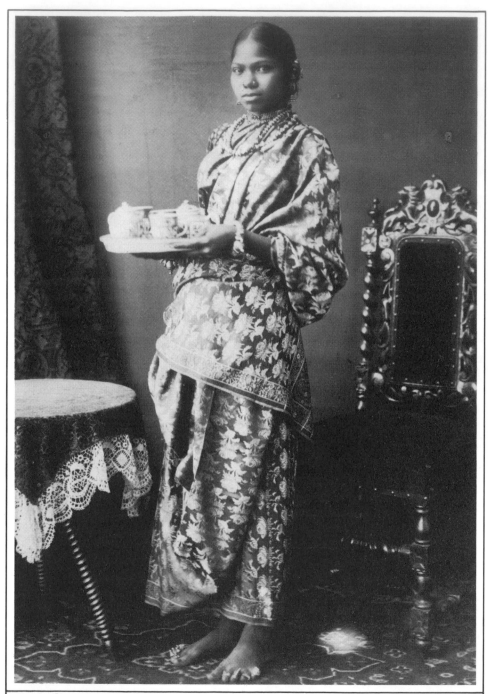

An Indian woman dressed in traditional clothing serves a pot of tea. Tea was first used in Asia as early as 4,700 years ago both as a social drink and for medicinal purposes.

USES AND ABUSES

JACK H. MENDELSON, M.D.
NANCY K. MELLO, Ph.D.
Alcohol and Drug Abuse Research Center
Harvard Medical School—McLean Hospital

*H*uman beings are endowed with the gift of wizardry, a talent for discovery and invention. The discovery and invention of substances that change the way we feel and behave are among our special accomplishments, and like so many other products of our wizardry, these substances have the capacity to harm as well as to help.

Consider alcohol—available to all and recognized as both harmful and pleasure inducing since biblical times. The use of alcoholic beverages dates back to our earliest ancestors. Alcohol use and misuse became associated with the worship of gods and demons. One of the most powerful Greek gods was Dionysus, lord of fruitfulness and god of wine. The Romans adopted Dionysus but changed his name to Bacchus. Festivals and holidays associated with Bacchus celebrated the harvest and the origins of life. Time has blurred the images of the Bacchanalian festival, but the theme of drunkenness as a major part of celebration has survived the pagan gods and remains a familiar part of modern society. The term *Bacchanalian festival* conveys a more appealing image than "drunken orgy" or "pot party," but whatever the label, some of the celebrants will inevitably start up the "high" escalator to the next plateau. Once there, the de-escalation is often difficult.

According to reliable estimates, 1 out of every 10 Americans develops a serious alcohol-related problem sometime in his or her lifetime. In addition, automobile accidents caused by drunken drivers claim the lives of more than 20,000 people each year, and injure 25 times that number. Many of the victims are gifted young people just starting out in adult life. Hospital emergency rooms abound with patients seeking help for alcohol-related injuries.

Who is to blame? Can we blame the many manufacturers who produce such an amazing variety of alcoholic beverages? Should we blame the educators who fail to explain the perils of intoxication or so exaggerate the dangers of drinking that no one could possibly believe them? Are friends to blame— those peers who urge others to "drink more and faster," or the macho types who stress the importance of being able to "hold your liquor?" Casting blame, however, is hardly constructive, and pointing the finger is a fruitless way to deal with problems. Alcoholism and drug abuse have few culprits but many victims. Accountability begins with each of us, every time we choose to use or to misuse an intoxicating substance.

It is ironic that some of our earliest medicines, derived from natural plant products, are used today to poison and to intoxicate. Relief from pain and suffering is one of society's many continuing goals. More than 3,000 years ago, the Therapeutic Papyrus of Thebes, one of our earliest written records, gave instructions for the use of opium in the treatment of pain. Opium, in the form of its major derivative, morphine, remains one of the most powerful drugs we have for pain relief. But opium, morphine, and similar compounds, such as heroin, have also been used by many to induce changes in mood and feeling. Another example of a natural substance that has been misused is the coca leaf, which for centuries was used by the Indians of Peru to reduce fatigue and hunger. Its modern derivative, cocaine, has important medical use as a local anesthetic. Unfortunately, its increasing abuse in recent years has reached epidemic proportions.

The purpose of this series is to provide information about the nature and behavioral effects of alcohol and drugs and the probable consequences of their use. The authors believe that up-to-date, objective information about alcohol and drugs will help readers make better decisions about the wisdom of their use. The information presented here (and in other books in this series) is based on many clinical and laboratory studies and observations by people from diverse walks of life.

Over the centuries, novelists, poets, and dramatists have provided us with many insights into the effects of alcohol and drug use. Physicians, lawyers, biologists, psychologists, and social scientists have contributed to a better understanding of the causes and consequences of using these substances. The authors in this series have attempted to gather and condense all the latest information about drug use. They have also described the sometimes wide gaps in our knowledge and have suggested some new ways to answer many difficult questions.

How, for example, do alcohol and drug problems get started? And what is the best way to treat them when they do? Not too many years ago, alcoholics and drug abusers were regarded as evil, immoral, or both. Many now believe that these persons suffer from very complicated diseases involving deep psychological and social problems. To understand how the disease begins and progresses, it is necessary to understand the nature of the substance, the behavior of the afflicted person, and the characteristics of the society or culture in which that person lives.

The diagram below shows the interaction of these three factors. The arrows indicate that the substance not only affects the user personally but the society as well. Society influences attitudes toward the substance, which in turn affect its availability. The substance's impact upon the society may support or discourage the use and abuse of that substance.

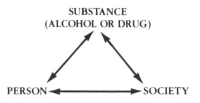

Although many of the social environments we live in are very similar, some of the most subtle differences can strongly influence our thinking and behavior. Where we live, go to school and work, whom we discuss things with—all influence our opinions about drug use. Yet we also share certain commonly accepted beliefs that outweigh any differences in our attitudes. The authors in this series have tried to identify and discuss the central, most crucial issues concerning drug use.

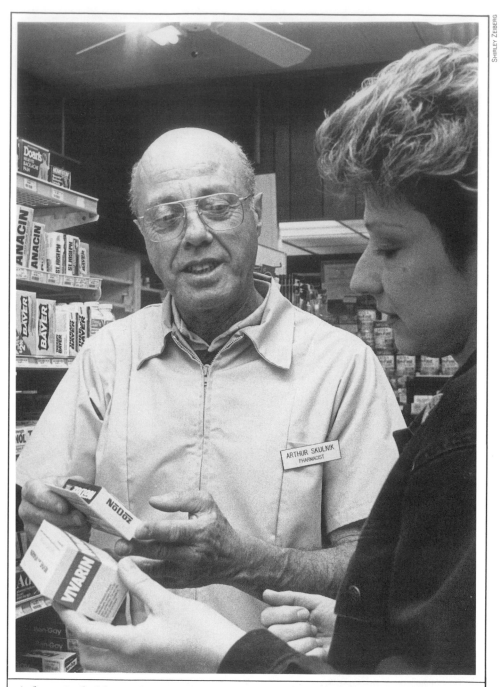

SHIRLEY ZEIBERG

A druggist holds packages of NoDoz and Vivarin, tablets sold without a prescription to promote alertness. The active ingredient in both of them is caffeine, which is also found in many other over-the-counter remedies for pain and other ailments.

Regrettably, human wizardry in developing new substances in medical therapeutics has not always been paralleled by intelligent usage. Although we do know a great deal about the effects of alcohol and drugs, we have yet to learn how to impart that knowledge, especially to young adults.

Does it matter? What harm does it do to smoke a little pot or have a few beers? What is it like to be intoxicated? How long does it last? Will it make me feel really fine? Will it make me sick? What are the risks? These are but a few of the questions answered in this series, which we hope will enable the reader to make wise decisions concerning the crucial issue of drugs.

Information sensibly acted upon can go a long way toward helping everyone develop his or her best self. As one keen and sensitive observer, Dr. Lewis Thomas, has said,

> *There is nothing at all absurd about the human condition. We matter. It seems to me a good guess, hazarded by a good many people who have thought about it, that we may be engaged in the formation of something like a mind for the life of this planet. If this is so, we are still at the most primitive stage, still fumbling with language and thinking, but infinitely capacitated for the future. Looked at this way, it is remarkable that we've come as far as we have in so short a period, really no time at all as geologists measure time. We are the newest, the youngest, and the brightest thing around.*

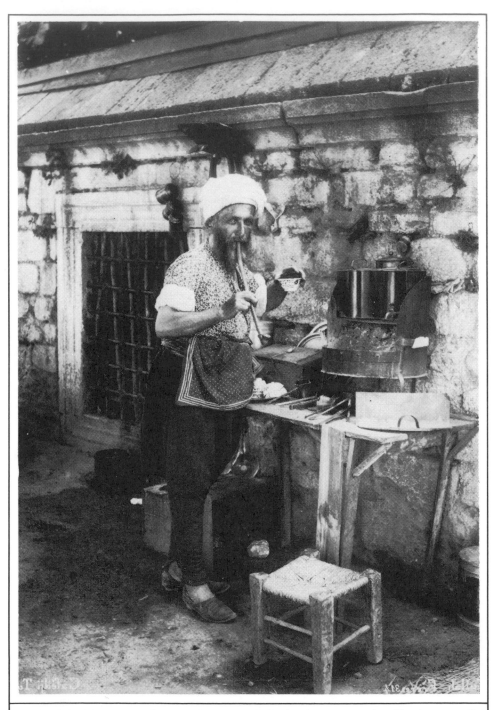

A Turk holds a cup of strong brew made by boiling ground coffee in one of the finjans, or small, long-handled pots, on the table.

CHAPTER 1

THE HISTORY OF TEA AND COFFEE

Caffeine, found naturally in coffee, tea, and chocolate, and as an additive in soft drinks and various medicinal remedies, is the most popular drug in the world. Caffeine a drug? Most people recognize two types of drugs. The first type includes chemicals such as aspirin and penicillin that can be purchased at the drugstore and are used to treat illnesses. And the second type includes substances such as heroin, cocaine, nicotine, and alcohol that people take to relax, to invigorate themselves, or to escape from reality.

Technically, a drug is a chemical substance used to prevent or cure disease or to enhance a person's physical or mental welfare. In fact, people use caffeine for all of these purposes and caffeine can do all of these things, though usually in a very limited way.

Though caffeine is a chemical used both for medical and nonmedical reasons, most often it is used nonmedically for its stimulating effect on mood and behavior. Drugs that are taken primarily to alter mood or change behavior are known as *psychoactive drugs*. Heroin, cocaine, marijuana, nicotine, alcohol, *and* caffeine are all psychoactive drugs.

Prehistory

Most of the known caffeine-yielding plants were probably discovered and used approximately 600,000 to 700,000 years ago, during the early Stone Age, or Paleolithic times. Paleolithic people chewed the seeds, bark, and leaves of many plants and they probably associated the chewing of parts of caffeine-containing plants with the resulting changes in mood and behavior. Eventually, caffeine was cultivated and consumed to banish fatigue, prolong wakefulness, and elevate mood.

Initially, Paleolithic people may have ground the caffeine-containing plant material to a paste and used it to aid digestion. Only much later was it discovered that by infusing

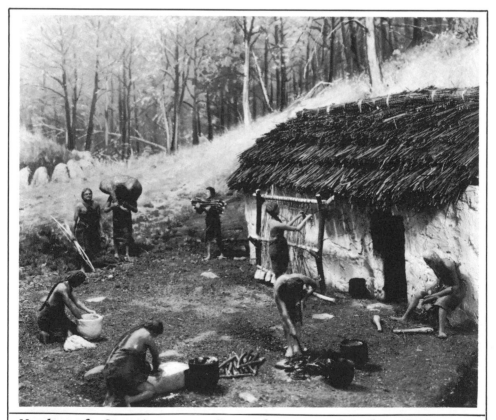

Members of a Stone Age community are shown at work in this artistic rendering of an early human settlement. Caffeine use has been traced as far back as Paleolithic times, at least 600,000 years ago.

the plant in hot water, a liquid could be created that when ingested produced greater effects. (This is true because more caffeine is extracted from a plant substance at higher temperatures.) This discovery led to the origin of all the caffeine-containing beverages, including maté, guarana, yoco infusion, cassina, kola tea, coffee, tea, and cocoa.

Tea

Tea has always been used both as a hot beverage and as a medicine. Records indicate that tea drinking may have existed in China as early as 4,700 years ago. Tea use and other aspects of Chinese culture spread to Japan around 600 C.E. (abbreviation for Common Era, equivalent to A.D.), but it took 700 years for it to become fully integrated into Japanese life. In

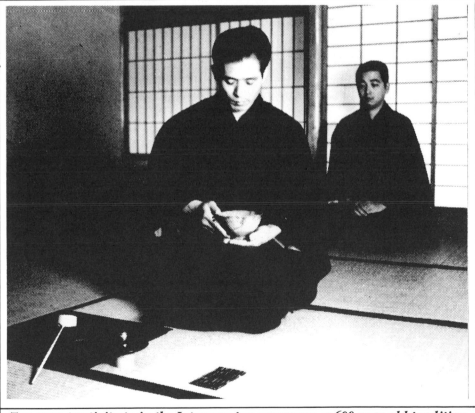

Two men participate in the Japanese tea ceremony, a 600-year-old tradition in which the serving and drinking of tea have become ritualized to create a sacred and aesthetic experience.

Japan tea became known by its Cantonese name, *ch'a*. In the 17th century, as the use of coffee was being introduced to Europe from Turkey, Dutch traders brought tea (originally called *tee*, from the Chinese Amoy dialect word *t'e*, pronounced "tay") back to their country. Despite its initial high cost, tea spread quickly throughout Europe and in some places displaced coffee as the beverage of choice.

Tea took a particularly strong hold in the North American colonies. American women were "such slaves to it," wrote one tourist in the 1760s, "that they would rather go without their dinners than without a dish of tea."

Partly to reaffirm its status as a strong colonial ruler, in 1767 the British government put a special tax on tea and several other items. As a result, the colonists boycotted tea and began using substitutes, particularly coffee. They were urged on by some local doctors and clergy, who attributed an assortment of ills and evils to tea drinking.

The tea boycott became a rallying point for the growing colonial independence movement. Colonists began destroying cargoes of tea in harbors along the East Coast. In Boston on December 16, 1773, a group of citizens disguised as In-

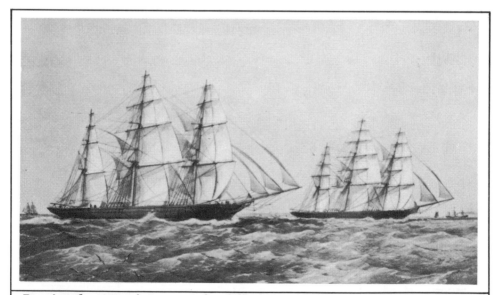

Bearing the season's tea crop for different companies, the clippers Taiping *and* Ariel *race each other from China to Britain in 1866 in this 19th century painting. The tea trade was highly competitive in the last century.*

dians boarded three moored ships and dumped their cargo of tea into the Boston harbor. This incident—the Boston Tea Party—and the British government's reprisals helped precipitate the American Revolution.

At first, the British did not realize the full significance of the Boston incident. Reports in London newspapers a month later focused not so much on the political implications of the event as on the effect of the tea on the unfortunate fish in the harbor. The fish, said one report, "had contracted a disorder not unlike the nervous complaints of the body." In fact, the large quantity of tea dumped into the harbor had given the fish a strong dose of caffeine.

At this time most tea came from China. Through the East India Company, the British had a near monopoly on the tea trade. When the company's commercial treaty with China

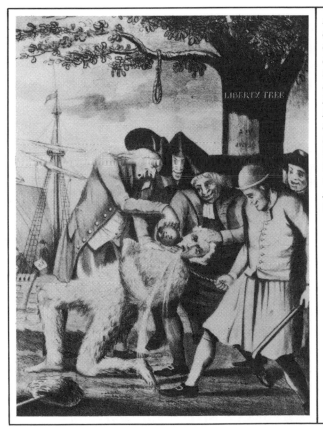

Patriotic colonists tar and feather a tax collector. The demonstration against the imposed tea tariff culminated with the Boston Tea Party on December 16, 1773, when a group of Bostonians, disguised as Indians, boarded a ship owned by the British East India Company and dumped 342 chests of tea into the harbor.

expired in 1833, however, the British control of the valuable tea trade became increasingly insecure. During the rest of the 19th century, tea plantations were developed in the Indian subcontinent. But China tea did not grow well in India, and the plantations became successful only when the local Assam variety of tea was cultivated. As recently as the 1870s more than 90% of Britain's tea still came from China.

The insecurity of Britain's hold on the tea trade was not helped by a domestic tax on tea that, in the early 19th century, was 15 times higher than the tax on coffee. As a consequence, coffee use in Britain increased tenfold between 1800 and 1840, at which time the beverage overtook tea in popularity. A series of coffee-adulteration scandals, however, led many people to return to tea. To the distress of buyers and drinkers, chicory, roasted corn, vegetable roots, and baked horse liver were discovered as having been used to increase the bulk of ground coffee. Also, in the mid-nineteenth century, the taxes on tea were lowered. Thus, tea once again became the beverage of choice for the British.

Another country in which tea has been extremely popular is Ireland, although Prime Minister Eamon De Valera attempted to ban the drink in the 1930s. In a symbolic effort to rid his country of British influence, which he claimed was preventing the full flowering of national aspiration, De Valera led the movement to ban tea by promoting indigenous milk and beer as alternatives. The campaign, however, was unsuccessful, and today Ireland remains the leading non-Arabian tea-drinking country in the world.

Coffee

The first written mention of coffee is found in Arabian documents of the 10th century. There is evidence, though, that in Ethiopia coffee was cultivated and the berries chewed as early as the 6th century. An Arabian legend tells of a young goatherd who discovered the stimulative effect of the berries after noticing that his goats became very frisky after grazing on coffee bushes. Coffee berries were still being chewed in tropical Africa in the 19th century. Before the Arabian peoples took to making a hot beverage from beans, they crushed them, fermented the juice, and made a wine called *qahwah*. When at the beginning of the 11th century they began to use the beans to produce the hot drink, they also called it *qah-*

wah. As use of the beverage spread throughout the world this word was adapted to the various languages of coffee-using people, producing such words as café, Kaffee, koffie, and coffee.

By the end of the 17th century the Dutch had established coffee plantations on the Indonesian island of Java. During the next 50 years, first the French and then the British followed suit in their Caribbean colonies. Commercial cultivation of coffee spread from the Caribbean to Central and South America, and by the early 19th century Brazil had supplanted Indonesia as the major producer and exporter of coffee. By 1860 the United States was consuming three-quarters of the world's coffee, more than half of which came from Brazil.

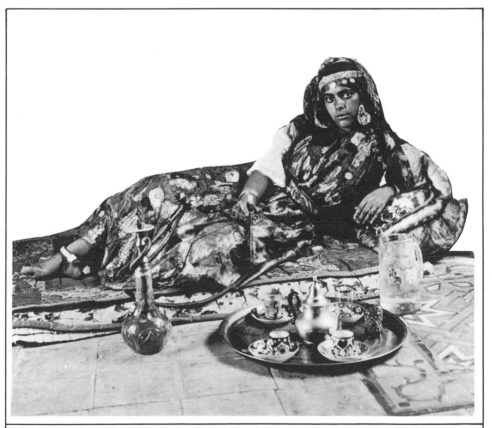

A Moorish woman lounges next to her water pipe and coffee. There is evidence that coffee berries were chewed in Africa as far back as the 6th century, 500 years before the hot drink was first produced.

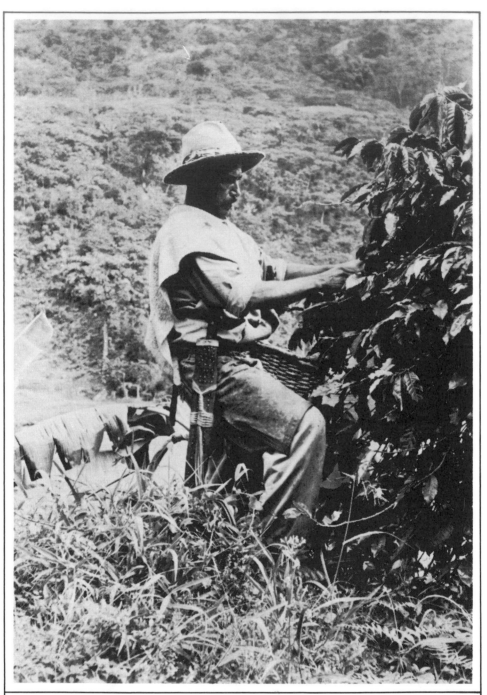

A coffee picker at work. In Colombia, berries are picked at optimum grades of ripeness, requiring the picker to return to the same tree several times during harvest and pick the red berries one at a time.

CHAPTER 2

SOURCES OF CAFFEINE

Nearly all of the approximately 120,000 tons of caffeine consumed in the world each year comes from coffee and tea plants. About 54% of this caffeine comes from coffee beans and 43% comes from tea leaves. The remaining 3% comes mostly from cacao pods, which are the basis of cocoa butter and chocolate, and also from kola nuts, maté leaves, and many other sources. Only a very small amount of caffeine is chemically synthesized in laboratories.

Not all of the caffeine derived from coffee and tea plants ends up in coffee mugs and tea cups. A considerable amount is extracted from low-quality coffee beans and tea leaves or is collected as a by-product of the decaffeination of coffee and tea. This caffeine is used in soft drinks and in medicines.

The beans used to produce coffee grow on only three species. *Coffea arabica*, native to Ethiopia, is now cultivated chiefly in Brazil and Colombia; *Coffea robusta*, native to Saudi Arabia, is now cultivated chiefly in Indonesia, Brazil, and many parts of Africa; and *Coffea liberica*, native to Liberia, is currently cultivated in Africa. Tea leaves used in brewing tea grow on a single species, *Camellia sinensis*, native to China and India where it is still chiefly cultivated. Wild species of both genuses grow abundantly—*Coffea* in Africa and *Camellia* in the Yunnan province of China, where a plant over 90 feet tall and 1,800 years old has been reported.

Table 1

Plant Sources of Caffeine					
SOURCE	PLANT PART	COUNTRY OF ORIGIN	CURRENT MAJOR CULTIVATION SITE	MEANS OF CAFFEINE INTAKE	TYPICAL CAFFEINE CONTENT (% weight)
Coffee bean					
Coffea arabica L.	seed	Ethiopia	Brazil, Colombia	coffee	1.1
Coffea robusta	seed	Arabia	Indonesia, Africa	coffee	2.2
Coffea liberica	seed	Liberia	Africa	coffee	1.4
Tea					
Camellia sinensis	leaf, bud	China	India, China	tea	3.5
Kola nut					
Cola acuminata S.	seed	West Africa	West Africa	chewing nuts kola tea	1.5
Cola nitida					
Cacao pod					
Theobroma cacao L.	seed	Mexico	West Africa, Brazil	cocoa and chocolate products	0.03 1.7
Maté					
Ilex paraquayensis	leaf	South America	South America	yerba maté	less than 0.7
Yaupon					
Ilex cassine	leaf, berry	North America	(not cultivated)	cassina	unknown
I. vomitoria					
Guarana paste					
Paullinia capana	seed	Brazil	Brazil	guarana bars and beverage	more than 4
P. sorbilis					
Yoco					
Paullinia yoco	bark	South America	South America	yoco infusion	2.7

SOURCE: G. A. Spiller, ed. *The Methylxanthine Beverages & Foods.* New York: Alan R. Liss, 1984.

The other commercially valuable plant sources of caffeine are cocoa beans and kola nuts, produced mainly in Africa, and maté leaves, guarana seeds, and yoco bark, all of which grow in South America. Only maté is consumed in any quantity, and then only in Paraguay, Uruguay, and Argentina. Table 1 summarizes the information about these major sources of caffeine. One should note that because tea is made with approximately four times as much water per weight as is coffee, a cup of coffee can contain considerably more caffeine than a cup of tea.

Why Plants Contain Caffeine

To understand why certain plants have evolved to contain caffeine, researchers have focused on how this chemical compound might benefit these plants. One idea is that caffeine-containing plants gain extra protection from attack by bacteria, fungi, and insects. Caffeine is known to inhibit the actions of bacteria and fungi, and to cause sterility in certain insects, which decreases the insect population. In addition, because caffeine gets into the surrounding soil, it may inhibit the growth of weeds that might otherwise destroy the plants. Obviously, a plant containing a substance that gives it this kind of protection will have a higher survival rate than one that either has a smaller amount or none at all.

However, if caffeine were to harm the plant itself this advantage would be lost. In fact, caffeine-containing plants do have mechanisms for protecting themselves against the caffeine's poisonous effects. For example, coffee plants produce and store the caffeine in coffee seedlings, away from the sites of cell division, which is very sensitive to toxic substances. But caffeine may still eventually kill the coffee plants that produced it. As a caffeine-bearing bush or tree

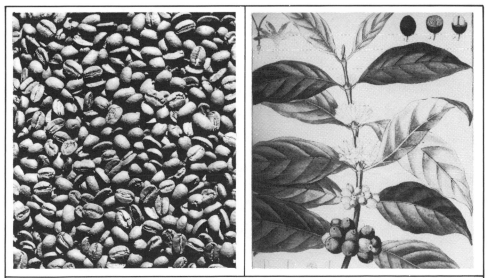

Roasted coffee beans (left) from Coffea arabica, *illustrated here with both ripe and immature berries. Cross-sections of two berries show that each one contains two coffee beans.*

ages, the soil around it becomes increasingly rich in caffeine that it has absorbed from the accumulation of the plant's fallen leaves and berries. It is partially because of this that coffee plantations tend to degenerate after 10 to 25 years.

Coffee Cultivation

Coffea arabica, which accounts for about 75% of all coffee consumption, is an evergreen tree or shrub that grows best in areas with moderate rainfall and at altitudes of between 2,000 feet and 6,500 feet above sea level. In Ecuador it is cultivated as high as 9,400 feet, while in subtropical Hawaii it is grown near the sea. It is also necessary for the temperature to remain as close as possible to 68°F. The variety that is cultivated commercially grows to a height of approximately 16 feet, though to ease harvesting it is frequently trimmed to a height of about 6 feet.

Three or four years after planting, *Coffea arabica* produces highly scented blossoms. The coffee berries ripen six to eight months later, changing from dark green to yellow, then to red, and eventually to deep crimson when they are fully ripe. Because of their size and general appearance, the ripe berries are known as coffee cherries. Beneath the crimson skin of the cherry is a moist, soft, sweet-tasting pulp that surrounds the green coffee bean. The bean itself has a thin, delicate, translucent covering known as the silver skin.

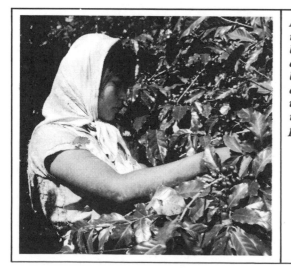

A woman picking coffee berries in Brazil. Because a tree can bear ripe and unripe berries at the same time, the ripe berries must be singled out and then picked by hand. A worker must pick 2000 berries in order to produce a single pound of roasted coffee.

The proper time to harvest varies according to climate and altitude. Where conditions are less than ideal, as in southern Brazil, coffee is harvested only in the winter. Under perfect conditions, as in Java, planting is staggered throughout the year, and therefore the coffee can be harvested almost continuously. The berries are picked by hand or shaken from the bush onto mats.

Coffea arabica is a delicate plant which is plagued by more than 40 diseases caused by fungi, viruses, bacteria, and soil deficiencies. The worst disease is leaf rust caused by the fungus Hemileia vastatrix. The leaves die and drop off, and after a few years the bush dies. Leaf rust damage is a problem almost everywhere except in Central and South America, where farmers destroy the plants at the first sign of the disease. This success in fighting leaf rust explains why most Arabica coffee is grown there. Other, less serious diseases do occur, but mostly where growing conditions are marginal.

Coffea robusta (also known as Coffea canephora var. robusta) is grown mostly outside the Americas, although some is grown in Brazil. It is more tolerant of extremes of soil and climate and more resistant to diseases and insects than is Coffea arabica. Coffea robusta will also grow at lower altitudes. C. robusta berries take from two or three months longer to ripen than do C. arabica berries, though they typically yield larger harvests. In addition, harvesting is easier because the C. robusta berries stay on the tree when they are overripe. These differences mean that it costs less to grow C. robusta coffee, and this cost difference accounts for the increasing use of this coffee plant, despite its reportedly inferior taste.

Coffee Processing

There are two methods used to separate the bean from the berry. In the *wet process*, a pulping machine breaks open the freshly picked berries and removes the skin and some of the flesh beneath. They are then left in water for about 24 hours, during which time more of the flesh is loosened by the action of yeasts and bacteria (fermentation). Afterwards, the beans are washed and then dried in the sun. Finally their silver skin is removed and they are machine polished. This yields what are known by coffee traders as *green beans*. This wet process, used for all Arabica coffee berries except for those in Brazil, generally produces a higher grade of bean.

Dry processing is a less expensive method of separating the bean from the berry and is used for almost all Robusta coffees and for Arabica coffees in Brazil. In this method the berries are stripped from the plant and either dried in special machines or left to dry in the sun for two to three weeks. After this period the dried husks and silver skins are readily removed by machinery or even by hand to yield the green coffee beans. Dry processing produces beans which create a harsher tasting coffee than those beans processed by the wet method. For this reason Arabica coffee from Brazil tends not to be of the highest quality. When *C. robusta* berries are wet processed, as they are in Uganda, the result is a bean that is better than most other Robustas.

Under the right conditions, green coffee beans may be stored for many years. They are usually exported in 60-kg bags (1 kg = 2.2 lbs.), although there is a large international trade in processed (soluble or instant) coffee.

Much of the coffee that is consumed undergoes further processing to produce decaffeinated coffee. Because some of

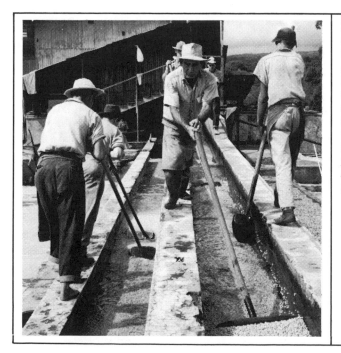

The wet process converts the coffee berry to ready-for-export green coffee beans. The beans, which have been depulped by machine, travel by sluiceway to the drying area. In these sluiceways, fresh water removes any substances that may be clinging to the beans.

the oils and other flavor components of the coffee bean are lost during the various processes, the stronger tasting Robustas and the dry-processed Arabicas from Brazil are generally used.

In an attempt to remove 97% or more of the caffeine, while leaving or returning to the bean as much of the flavor components as possible, manufacturers use two primary techniques, the *direct method* and the *water method.* In the direct method, a chemical solvent, methylene chloride, is used to remove caffeine from the green beans; the solvent is then mixed with water and the caffeine is extracted for other uses. In the water method, the green beans are soaked in water; after the caffeine is removed from this water, the beans are once again returned to the water in an attempt to restore some of their flavor-retaining solids. Decaffeinated coffee produced by the direct method is generally superior in flavor to that produced by the water method, which removes most of the body and flavor along with the caffeine. However, consumers continue to express concern about the safety of decaffeinated coffee produced by the direct method, despite an announcement by the U.S. Food and Drug Administration in

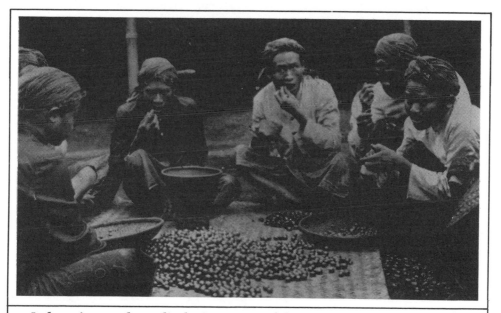

Indonesian workers, displaying a type of dry processing, crack the coffee berry open with their teeth in order to remove the coffee beans.

1985 that the risk from using methylene chloride in decaffeination is virtually nonexistent; according to the FDA, the amount left in coffee after processing is minute, no greater than that found in the air of many cities. In the late 1980s scientists devised a new direct process for caffeine extraction, employing carbon dioxide instead of methylene chloride; this new method is said to result in a more flavorful beverage because it removes only the caffeine, not the flavorful solids. In 1990 it was being used by two manufacturers of caffeine-free coffee in the United States.

Roasting of both regular and decaffeinated green beans is generally carried out shortly before they reach the retail market. This is done commercially by passing the green beans through 260°C gases for up to 5 minutes, the length of roasting time depending on the desired darkness of the bean which in turn affects the taste and caffeine content of the brewed coffee. The bean loses water during roasting—14% during the shortest roast, known as "light city," which produces a cinnamon-colored bean, and 20% during the longest roast, known as "Italian," which produces a dark brown to black bean. The final step before brewing is grinding, which is usually done by the processor or in the store, but increasingly it is

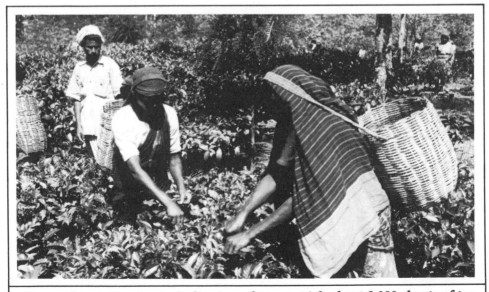

Women harvesting tea in India. A worker can pick about 3,000 shoots of tea a day, which produces less than one pound of manufactured tea.

being done at the point of preparation in homes or restaurants so that no flavor is lost.

Instant coffee is produced from the roasted beans using one of two methods. Both begin by brewing a coffee extract in huge percolators. Pressurized water at 338°F is used to force more of the bean into solution. In the manufacture of *spray-dried coffee* the extract is fed into the top of a tower of hot air. This dries the extract into a powder, which can be recovered from the bottom of the tower. *Freeze-dried coffee*, more expensive though better tasting, takes advantage of the fact that the water and the solids in the coffee extract separate upon freezing. Afterwards the solids are granulated or turned into flakes.

Tea Cultivation

The tea plant, *Camellia sinensis*, has a great number of varieties, or subspecies. Considerable confusion once existed as to whether there was one or more species of the plant, but in 1958 it was internationally agreed that there is one species with several varieties, of which two have major commercial importance.

Like the coffee plant, the tea plant is an evergreen tree or bush that grows in the tropics or subtropics. It grows best at altitudes of between 2,000 and 6,500 feet and in areas that

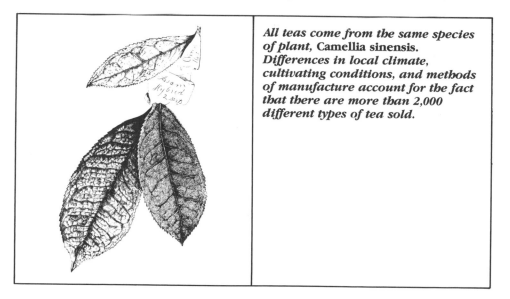

All teas come from the same species of plant, Camellia sinensis. *Differences in local climate, cultivating conditions, and methods of manufacture account for the fact that there are more than 2,000 different types of tea sold.*

receive moderate rainfall. The most cultivated variety is Assam tea, or var. *assamica*, which because of its low resistance
to cold survives best in tropical areas. China tea, or var. *sinensis*, has lower yields than Assam tea but produces a more
delicately flavored beverage. It can tolerate brief cold periods
and thus higher altitudes than Assam tea. In the 1800s China
tea was cultivated in South Carolina, but the plantations
were abandoned because high labor costs made them eco-
nomically unsound. However, many plants still survive in this
area.

The Assam tea plant has large leaves, up to 10 inches
long, and if left uncultivated can grow to a height of 50 feet.
The China tea plant is smaller, with 4-inch leaves and a natural
height of no more than 20 feet. Both plants are trimmed to
waist height to facilitate plucking of the leaves. Ideally, only
young leaves and shoots are harvested. Plucking only the
young leaves in such a way as to keep the plant healthy is a
highly skilled job. Though to reduce labor costs mechanical
shearing is on the increase, this method produces a coarse
tea of varying quality.

Tea Processing

After plucking, the leaves are most frequently treated in one
of two ways. About three-quarters of the leaves destined for
beverage use are made into *black tea*; the other quarter becomes *green tea*, the type generally served in Asian restaurants. Because of the type of equipment required, the
manufacture of black tea is carried out almost exclusively in
large factories. Green tea can be produced under the small-
scale conditions of the family farm, though today it is most
frequently manufactured on a larger scale. To produce black
tea, freshly plucked leaves are withered and then squeezed
or minced to release their sap. The sap contains the enzyme
(an organic catalyst) *tea polyphenol oxidase*, which causes
the plant's colorless flavor-producing chemicals to take up
oxygen from the air. This oxidizing process changes the
leaves' character and in addition turns them dark brown.

To produce green tea, the oxidizing enzyme is destroyed
before it can cause changes in color and flavor. This is done
by heat—steam heat in Japan and dry heat in China. Because
it contains unoxidized flavor-producing substances, green tea
tends to have a more bitter flavor than black tea. After this

initial step is completed, the leaves are treated much as black tea. Both teas contain a similar amount of caffeine.

After manufacture, the tea is sorted by size, purged of stalks and dust, packed in foil-lined chests, and shipped to blenders or auctioneers. Each chest contains between 30 kg and 60 kg of tea leaf. In North America, more than 90% of tea is packaged in the form of tea bags.

A small portion of the tea is further processed to remove the caffeine or to produce instant tea. The decaffeination of tea is very similar to the decaffeination of coffee, most often utilizing the same solvent, methylene chloride, to extract the caffeine from the moistened leaf.

Instant tea is also manufactured in a manner similar to that of instant coffee. First, an extract is prepared by subjecting the leaves to high-temperature and high-pressure water. Then the extract is spray-dried to produce a powder. Since most instant tea is used to make iced tea, further processing may be required to ensure that the powder is soluble in cold water. Prior to marketing, the tea powder is often blended with a sweetener and/or lemon flavoring.

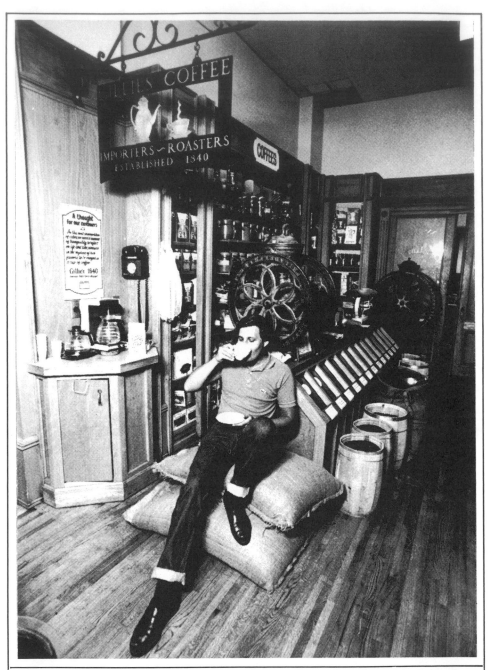

The owner of a coffee store in New York City takes a break amidst barrels and bins of coffee, coffeemakers, and grinders. Although most coffee sold in the United States is ground by the manufacturer prior to sale, increasing numbers of coffee drinkers are grinding the beans as they need them in order to produce a fresher-flavored beverage.

CHAPTER 3

CAFFEINE CONSUMPTION TODAY

*T*he amount of caffeine in cups of coffee and tea varies enormously (see Table 2). Excluding decaffeinated coffees and teas, the range for a six-ounce cup of coffee is from 40 mg to about 150 mg and the range for a similar amount of tea is from 20 mg to as much as 90 mg. This wide variance is mainly due to the quantity and quality of the coffee bean or tea leaf used, as well as the method of preparation. Because of this it can be very difficult to compare two people's caffeine intake by simply asking them how many cups of coffee or cups of tea they drink.

Drip coffee contains more caffeine than percolated coffee, which in turn contains more caffeine than instant coffee. The large difference in caffeine content between drip and percolated coffee found in home-prepared beverages is probably an indication that more coffee bean per cup was used to make drip coffee. In making drip coffee the water passes over the ground bean only once, while in a percolator it repeatedly passes over the ground bean. In fact, nearly all of the caffeine is dissolved in the near-boiling water during the first pass, especially if the bean is ground finely. Repeated passing only causes more of the other coffee bean components to go into solution. These other components add to the bitterness of the beverage, and thus its apparent strength, though the caffeine content is only very minimally affected. To decrease the bitterness, people tend to use less bean when percolating coffee.

Table 2

Amounts of Caffeine in Common Beverages, Foods, and Drugs	
	Milligrams of caffeine
Coffee (6-ounce cup, drip method)	110-150
Instant coffee (6-ounce cup)	40-108
Decaffeinated coffee (6-ounce cup, brewed)	2-5
Tea (6-ounce cup, 3-minute brew)	20-46
Hot cocoa (6-ounce cup)	2-8
Sweet dark chocolate (1 ounce)	5-35
Coca-Cola (12-ounce can)	45.6
Diet Coke (12-ounce can)	45.6
Pepsi-Cola (12-ounce can)	38.4
No-Doz (1 tablet)	100
Vivarin (1 tablet)	200
Anacin (1 tablet)	32
Excedrin (1 tablet)	65

Source: Institute of Food Technologists

The variation in the caffeine content of home-prepared cups of tea is even greater than that for coffee. The variables here are the amount of tea leaf used (or the size of the tea bag), and the time the tea is left to brew. Caffeine is released from tea leaves a little more slowly than from coffee beans, especially if the leaves are in tea bags.

Caffeine is a constituent not only of cups of coffee and tea, including iced tea, but also of foods and beverages that are flavored with coffee or tea.

Caffeine in Soft Drinks

In addition to coffee and tea, a third major source of caffeine is soft drinks (see Table 2). In fact, given the decline in both coffee and tea consumption in the United States since 1960, more Americans are probably getting caffeine from cola-containing beverages than from any other source. In 1989 the five leading brands of soft drinks sold in the United States— Coke Classic, Pepsi, Diet Coke, Diet Pepsi, and Dr. Pepper— contained caffeine; together with Mountain Dew, ranked seventh in sales, caffeine-containing soft drinks accounted for an estimated 61% of the total (see Table 3). Although sales of

Table 3

Leading U.S. Soft Drink Brands and Their Caffeine Content				
	Market share, in percent			Caffeine content
Brand	1987	1988	E1989	(mg/12 oz.)
1. Coke Classic	19.8	20.1	20.0	45.6
2. Pepsi	18.8	18.7	18.3	38.4
3. Diet Coke	7.7	8.2	8.9	45.6
4. Diet Pepsi	4.8	5.2	5.7	38.4
5. Dr Pepper	4.3	4.5	4.6	40.0
6. Sprite	3.5	3.6	3.6	-
7. Mountain Dew	2.9	3.2	3.5	54.0
8. 7Up	3.4	3.1	2.9	-
9. Caffeine-free Diet Coke	1.7	2.0	2.4	-
10. Caffeine-free Diet Pepsi	1.3	1.4	1.5	-
Total	68.2	70.0	71.4	
E=Estimated				

Source: *Beverage Digest;* Soft Drink Manufacturers Association

caffeine-free beverages, particularly colas, continue to increase, they are still a small percentage of the total. The top caffeine-free soft drink since the mid-1980s, Diet Caffeine-Free Coke, has a current market share of less than 3%.

More than 95% of the caffeine in soft drinks is added during manufacture. The remainder comes from the kola nut, the ingredient for which cola drinks were named when they were first introduced in the 1880s. At that time, Coca-Cola, the first of the colas, also contained cocaine, which occurs naturally in coca leaves. Since 1903 the coca leaves used in the manufacture of colas have been decocainized, although manufacturers have not been required to demonstrate the absence of cocaine since 1969. Today, Coke probably contains very small amounts of cocaine.

Caffeine in Cocoa and Chocolate

Cocoa and chocolate products are other major sources of caffeine (see Tables 2 and 4). The range of caffeine content in these products varies considerably, although the caffeine content of these products is relatively low. Only chocolate bars contain a significant amount of caffeine, and here the range is also great. Only the finest quality sweet, or dark, chocolate has a high caffeine content. The typical 50-gram (ca. 1.6 oz.) milk chocolate bar sold in North America has about 10 mg of caffeine if it is mostly chocolate, and much less if there is a substantial quantity of nonchocolate filler such as nuts and fudge, or if some or all of the chocolate is artificial.

The theobromine content of each item is also given in Table 4. As previously mentioned, theobromine is similar to caffeine in structure and effect on the body, though it is only one-tenth as potent. However, cocoa and chocolate products typically have approximately 10 times as much theobromine as caffeine. Therefore, the caffeine-like effects produced by consuming a cocoa or chocolate product may be about twice as great as the effects one might expect from the actual caffeine content.

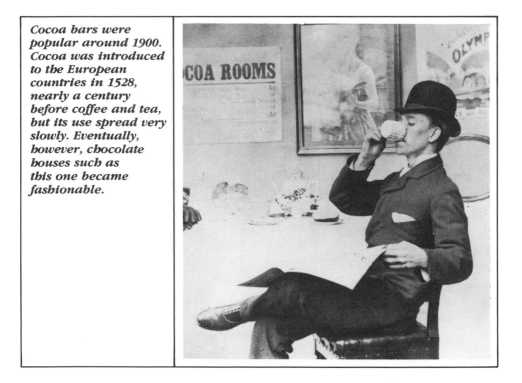

Cocoa bars were popular around 1900. Cocoa was introduced to the European countries in 1528, nearly a century before coffee and tea, but its use spread very slowly. Eventually, however, chocolate houses such as this one became fashionable.

Table 4

Caffeine and Theobromine Content of Cocoa and Chocolate Products

PRODUCT	SERVING SIZE	CAFFEINE (mg)	THEOBROMINE (mg)
Chocolate bar	50 grams (1.6 oz.)	3-63	68-314
Hot cocoa	150 milliliters (5 oz.)	1-8	40-80
Chocolate milk	225 milliliters (7.6 oz.)	2-7	35-99
Chocolate-chip cookie	30 grams (ca. 1 oz.)	3-5	21-30
Chocolate ice cream	50 grams (1.6 oz.)	2-5	15-39

Source: G. A. Spiller, ed. *The Methylxanthine Beverages & Foods*. New York: Alan R. Liss, 1984.

Caffeine in Medicines

Caffeine is added to many prescription drugs, most commonly to remedies for migraine headaches (Cafergot, for example) and other forms of pain (Darvon, Fiorinal). It is also an ingredient in numerous over-the-counter stimulants, pain relievers, and diet drugs; Table 2 includes the caffeine content per tablet of several popular OTC stimulants and painkillers.

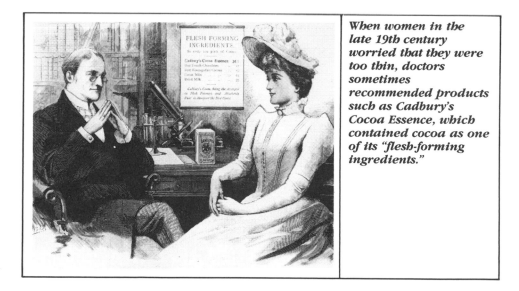

When women in the late 19th century worried that they were too thin, doctors sometimes recommended products such as Cadbury's Cocoa Essence, which contained cocoa as one of its "flesh-forming ingredients."

Table 5

Coffee Consumption in the United States (Cups per Person per Day)				
	1962	1972	1982	1989
All Coffee	3.12	2.25	1.90	1.75
Types:				
Regular	2.45	1.67	1.33	1.43
Instant	0.67	0.68	0.56	0.32
Decaffeinated*	0.10	0.17	0.38	0.40
Region:				
North-East	2.91	2.10	1.85	1.79
North-Central	3.34	2.66	2.18	1.98
South	2.78	1.97	1.68	1.52
West	3.52	2.74	1.96	1.81
Age Groups:				
10-14	0.18	0.12	0.03	0.02
15-19	1.09	0.55	0.33	0.20
20-24	2.99	1.48	0.92	0.72
25-29	3.88	2.47	1.75	1.23
30-39	4.50	3.51	2.37	2.03
40-49	4.44	3.72	3.11	2.65
50-59	3.83	3.35	3.09	2.97
60-69	3.01	2.85	2.55	2.64
70 and over	2.39	2.49	2.03	1.93
Sex:				
Male	3.28	2.48	2.06	1.85
Female	2.98	2.23	1.75	1.66
Location:				
Home	2.57	1.86	1.36	1.23
Work	0.26	0.28	0.38	0.34
Eating Places	0.29	0.21	0.14	0.18
Time of Day:				
Breakfast	1.17	1.00	0.88	0.90
Other Meals	0.98	0.59	0.36	0.22
Between Meals	0.97	0.76	0.66	0.63
Cups per Drinker per Day	4.17	c. 3.7	3.38	3.34
Percentage of Population Drinking Coffee	74.7	c. 63.0	56.3	52.5

*Decaffeinated coffee is not separate from regular and instant but is included in both types.

Source: Coffee Drinking Study, International Coffee Organization, 1989

Why caffeine is included in all these drugs is discussed in greater detail in Chapter 8.

Trends in Caffeine Beverage Use

Considerable changes have occurred in consumer preferences for caffeine-containing beverages in the United States since 1962. In that year the highest per-capita level of coffee consumption in the modern era was reached—3.12 cups per person per day. By 1972 that level had fallen to 2.25 cups, and in 1989 it stood at 1.75 cups. (See Table 5.) Although some of this decline can be attributed to concerns about the safety of coffee drinking, most of it had already occurred by the early 1970s, before the hazards of coffee use were widely publicized. On the other hand, decaffeinated coffee consumption, which has quadrupled since 1962, saw most of its growth occur between 1972 and 1982, and may thus reflect

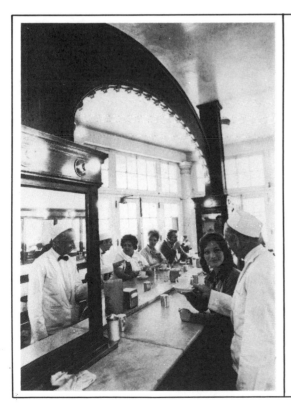

The decrease in coffee consumption in the United States since the 1960s is one factor in the decline of such establishments as the Morning Call Coffee Shop, which moved in 1983 from its location in the New Orleans French Quarter, where it had been for the past 103 years, to a suburb on the outskirts of the city.

the growing public concern during that period with the effects on health of caffeine. Decaffeinated coffee consumption still remains low, however: in 1989 the average per capita daily intake was less than half a cup.

The most striking differences in trends in coffee use have been among the age groups. The decline in use has been greatest in the youngest age group. It seems that coffee has become a drink for older people.

Because fewer young people are drinking coffee, use in the United States will most likely continue to decrease. The coffee industry's challenge is to change the non-coffee-drinking habits of what one coffee-industry executive recently has called "a young generation who finds coffee irrelevant to their lives except for an occasional wake-up cup. . . . [There is] a perception among young adults that coffee is for old, tired, frazzled, uninteresting, unsexy people."

Paralleling the decline in coffee consumption is the increasing consumer preference for soft drinks. Between 1960 and 1982 soft drink consumption grew an astonishing 230%, and from 1982 to 1989 it increased another 74%. Annual consumption per person is now about 48 gallons, which works out to 512 12 oz. servings, or almost 1½ cans per day. As noted earlier, caffeine-containing soft drinks currently account for some 61% of total consumption. Since each human being takes in a total of approximately 130 gallons of liquid, soft drinks now account for more than one-third of that total. For young people, this figure is considerably more than one-third. Children and teenagers consume half of all soft drinks, and the soft-drink habit appears to be persisting as they mature.

Ranges in Caffeine-Beverage Use

Each day Americans ingest on the average the equivalent of a cup and a half of medium-strength coffee and almost a serving each of tea and cola. However, few people fit this average exactly, in caffeine use or very much else. In reality there is a wide range of consumption of each of the caffeine-containing beverages. In the case of coffee, the reported range is from zero (people who drink no coffee) to the five or more cups per day consumed by heavy coffee drinkers.

The estimates of recent distributions of caffeine con-

Table 6

Distribution of Caffeine Use*	
RANGE OF CAFFEINE CONSUMPTION (mg/day)	% OF POPULATION
less than 50	15
50–200	40
200–350	25
350 500	12
600–650	5
more than 650	3

*North Americans aged 15 years and older

SOURCE: Author's personal data.

sumption among North Americans aged 15 and over are given in Table 6. These data take into account a number of changes in caffeine use that have occurred since the early 1970s, notably the fall in coffee use in the United States and the increase in use of caffeinated soft drinks. Some authorities have suggested that many more adults are using large amounts of caffeine. One such person wrote, "It is estimated that 30% of us take in 500 to 600 mg of caffeine per day, and 10%, more than 1,000 mg per day."

Given the fact that physical dependence on caffeine can occur when daily consumption of caffeine is in excess of about 350 mg (see Chapter 9), these data indicate that 20% of North American adults may be dependent on this substance. And since regular use of more than about 650 mg of caffeine a day can pose a risk to health (see Chapter 10), 3% of North Americans adults may be in danger.

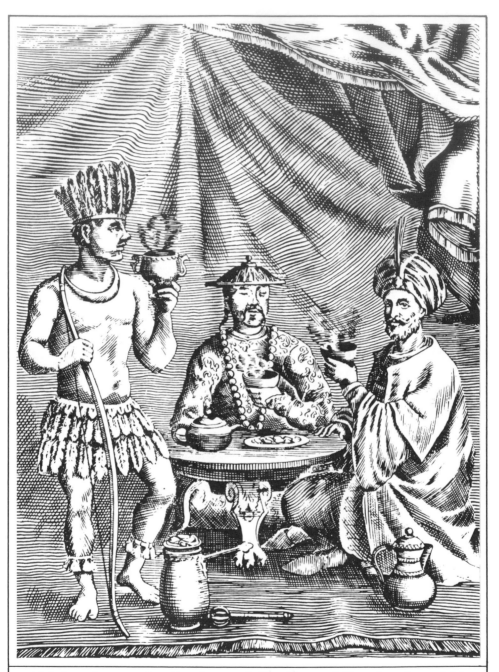

A 1688 French engraving, Treatises on Coffee, Tea, and Chocolate. *By weight tea leaves have more than twice as much caffeine as coffee beans, but a cup of coffee can have up to seven times more of the drug because more beans are used in the brew. Though cocoa has a much lower amount of caffeine, it contains large amounts of the stimulant theobromine.*

CHAPTER 4

THE CHEMISTRY OF CAFFEINE

Pure caffeine is a bitter-tasting white powder that resembles cornstarch. It is moderately soluble in water at body temperature and readily soluble in boiling water. It was first isolated from coffee in 1820 and from tea in 1827 and given the name *theine*. Soon thereafter it was recognized that the mood- and behavior-altering properties of both coffee and tea depended upon caffeine.

Caffeine has two technical names. The full name is 3,7-dihydro-1,3,7-trimethyl-1H-purine-2,6-dione. The more commonly used technical name is 1,3,7-trimethylxanthine. Both names describe the chemical structure of the caffeine molecule, whose two-dimensional representation is shown in Figure 1. Its chemical formula is $C_8H_{10}N_4O_2$.

To understand caffeine's effects, a brief introduction to purine and its related compounds is necessary (see Figure 1). Purine is the parent compound of all of these chemicals and of many other of the important chemicals found in the body. Upon closer inspection it can be seen that xanthine, or *dioxy*purine, is purine with two oxygen atoms, and that caffeine, or *trimethyl*xanthine, is xanthine with three methyl groups. As shown, a methyl group consists of a carbon atom and three hydrogen atoms. The "1,3,7" in caffeine's technical names refers to the positions of the methyl groups, as numbered in the purine structure.

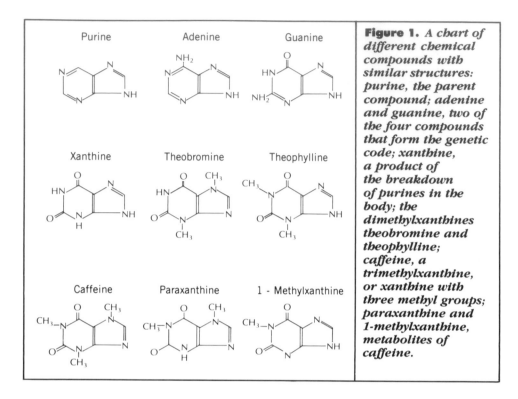

Figure 1. *A chart of different chemical compounds with similar structures: purine, the parent compound; adenine and guanine, two of the four compounds that form the genetic code; xanthine, a product of the breakdown of purines in the body; the dimethylxanthines theobromine and theophylline; caffeine, a trimethylxanthine, or xanthine with three methyl groups; paraxanthine and 1-methylxanthine, metabolites of caffeine.*

Purine does not occur in the body in its pure form. When chemicals in the purine family are broken down, xanthine is produced as an intermediate product. The liver further converts xanthine into uric acid, which is found in unusually high levels in humans. Though too much uric acid is associated with the disease known as gout, uric acid is believed to contribute to our living longer than most other mammals.

The two most important purines found in the body are adenine and guanine. These two, together with cytosine and thymine, comprise the four basic letters of the genetic alphabet, or code, found in the cells of all living organisms. Everything a person inherits—from membership in the human species to eye color—is determined by this code. The code is "read" in groups of three purines, each chemically bound to a long strand of molecules. Two strands and their purines make up what is called a DNA, or deoxyribonucleic acid, double helix. Genes are sequences of the groups of three purines found at specific places on the chromosomes, structures composed of DNA (see Figure 2).

The duplication of DNA is one of the central processes in the reproduction of cells and whole organisms. Caffeine, because of its similarity to critical parts of the genetic code, can interfere with this process and cause errors in the cells' reproduction. This may result in tumors, cancers, and genetic defects. The significance of caffeine's effects on reproduction is discussed further in Chapter 10.

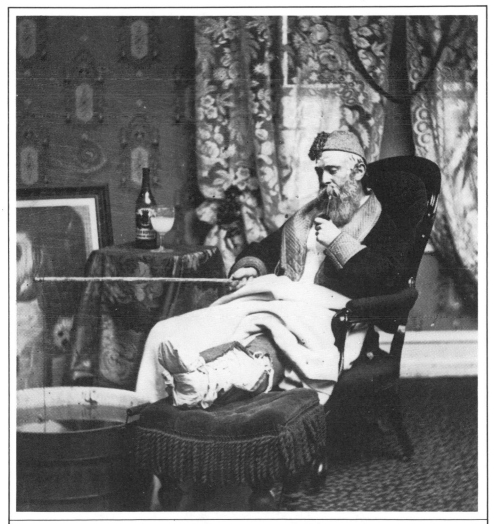

A person suffering from gout, a disease marked by painful swelling of the joints. Gout is caused by a high level of uric acid in the body, produced by the liver's breakdown of purines such as caffeine.

Theobromine and Theophylline

Theobromine and theophylline are two dimethylxanthines, or xanthine molecules, that have two rather than three methyl groups (see Figure 1). Both dimethylxanthines produce effects similar to caffeine's, though theobromine is considerably weaker, having no more than one-tenth of the stimulating effect of caffeine or theophylline.

Theobromine is found in cocoa products, tea (only in very small amounts), and kola nuts, but is not found in coffee. In cocoa, theobromine's concentration is generally about seven times as great as caffeine's. Because of this, although the caffeine content of cocoa products is relatively low, the actual caffeine-like effects produced by consuming these products will still be significant.

Theophylline, found in very small amounts with caffeine and theobromine in tea, may have a stronger stimulatory effect than caffeine on the heart and on breathing. It is often the drug of choice in treating diseases in which breathing is difficult, such as asthma, bronchitis, and emphysema. The theophylline used in medicine is made from caffeine extracted from coffee or tea.

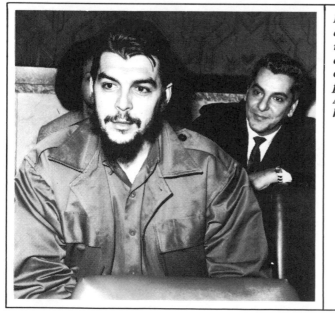

Ernesto "Che" Guevara, a well-known revolutionary leader, drank yerba maté, *a caffeine-rich beverage popular in Latin America, to ease his asthma.*

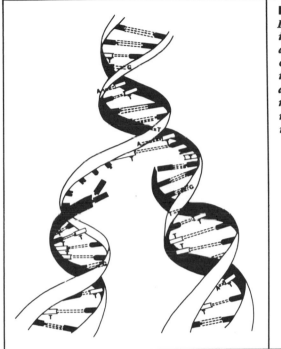

Figure 2. *An illustration of the DNA molecule. Because caffeine is similar in structure to adenine and guanine, two critical parts of the genetic code, it can interfere with the duplication of DNA and cause mutations, or errors, in cell reproduction, which can result in genetic defects.*

The Body's Absorption of Caffeine

Caffeine is moderately soluble in water and therefore can be found in the body wherever there is water—which is in most places. Caffeine also readily passes through cell membranes. Because of these properties, after caffeine is ingested it is rapidly and completely absorbed from the stomach and intestines into the bloodstream, which distributes it to all organs of the body, including the brain, the ovaries, and the testes. In addition, when a pregnant woman consumes a caffeine-containing food, the drug quickly goes to all of the organs of the unborn child.

In the bloodstream caffeine finally travels to the liver, where, by a process known as *metabolism*, it is converted into a number of breakdown products known as *metabolites*, which are eventually excreted in the urine. These metabolites include theobromine, theophylline, and a third dimethylxanthine, known as paraxanthine (see Figure 1).

Relatively high levels of paraxanthine are found in the blood after caffeine has been ingested. However, as the blood

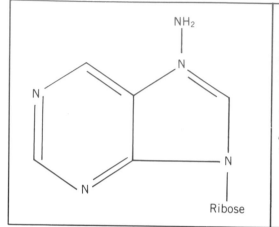

NH_2

N

N

N

N

Ribose

Figure 3. *The chemical adenosine (left) binds to receptor sites on the cell surface and thus inhibits the release of neurotransmitters, which causes sleepiness. Because of caffeine's structural similarity to adenosine, it can block adenosine's effects by binding to the receptor sites first and stimulating the neurotransmitters.*

passes through the liver again, paraxanthine is itself broken down to 1-methylxanthine (see Figure 1). Methylxanthine is the main metabolite of caffeine found in human urine, but typically it accounts for only about one-fifth of the caffeine dose. The remainder is turned into one of at least a dozen other products of caffeine metabolism.

Because caffeine so readily passes in both directions across membranes, it is not easily excreted by the kidneys into urine. If caffeine were not metabolized to compounds such as 1-methylxanthine that do not pass back across the kidney membrane and into the bloodstream, the caffeine from a cup of coffee would stay in the body for several days.

Frequently the metabolites of a drug have more effect than the drug that was originally ingested. Paraxanthine and, especially, 1-methylxanthine are even more similar to adenine and guanine than caffeine itself. Though it is not yet known exactly how much caffeine's metabolites contribute to caffeine's effects, both paraxanthine and 1-methylxanthine may very well play an important part in this drug's stimulation of the nervous system.

Caffeine's Effects

Caffeine's stimulatory effects involve the action of adenosine, a chemical widespread in the body (see Figure 3). The adenosine molecule, composed of a purine linked to a type of sugar, is part of a larger molecule that supplies energy necessary for all cell functions.

Adenosine is also an important regulator of body processes, particularly the transmission of signals by nerves. Injection of adenosine or substances that increase adenosine levels can cause lethargy and sleep. Adenosine can also dilate blood vessels, diminish gastrointestinal motility (the gastrointestinal organs' ability to contract), protect against seizures, retard the body's reaction to stress, and lower heart rate, blood pressure, and body temperature.

Adenosine inhibits the release of neurotransmitters, or chemicals that carry messages from one nerve cell to another. To do this it must first bind to specific receptor sites on the cell surface. Because its structure is so similar to adenosine's, caffeine also binds to the receptors, and, in doing so, caffeine prevents adenosine from binding there. Thus, the nerve cells fire more rapidly. Researchers have discovered that both paraxanthine and 1-methylxanthine are even more effective than caffeine in competing with adenosine for adenosine receptors. Therefore, caffeine's brain-stimulating effects may be enhanced by its being metabolized to paraxanthine and 1-methylxanthine.

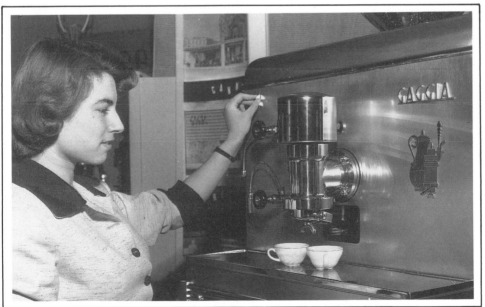

UPI/BETTMANN ARCHIVE

A visitor to a Milan industrial fair in 1955 serves herself coffee from the world's first automatic espresso machine, introduced that year.

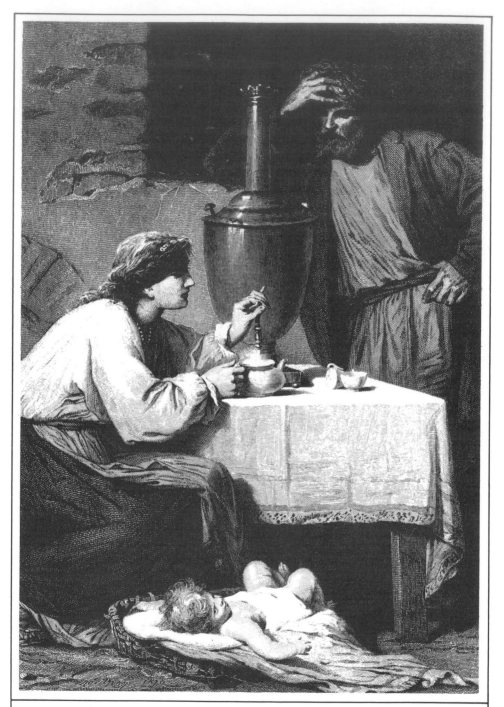

Tea-drinking rituals differ around the world. The woman in this Russian engraving, for example, is drawing the beverage from a samovar.

CHAPTER 5

CAFFEINE IN THE BODY

*D*rugs such as caffeine that affect behavior and mood usually do so by acting on some of the 50 billion nerve cells in the brain. To reach the brain the molecules of a drug must first get into the bloodstream, which they do by a process known as *absorption*. This is accomplished in two basic ways. In *enteral administration*, caffeine's most common form of ingestion, the route includes the gastrointestinal tract—the mouth, throat, stomach, intestines, and rectum.

Parenteral administration bypasses the gastrointestinal tract. Instead, the drug gets into the body via the lungs, skin, ear, or vagina, or by injection. Injections can be made directly into an artery or vein, into a muscle, into the spinal cord, or into some of the body's spaces, such as just under the skin or around the intestines. Though perhaps infrequently, caffeine has been administered through most of these routes.

Injection directly into the bloodstream is obviously the fastest route, but it is often the most dangerous. Some drugs, such as insulin, are not given enterally because they are destroyed by substances in the gastrointestinal tract. Other drugs, such as some of the barbiturates, cannot pass from the gastrointestinal tract into the blood vessels in the wall of the stomach and intestines. Therefore, these drugs are also not given enterally. And because the blood from the stomach and intestines goes to the liver before going to the brain, drugs such as cocaine and heroin, which are broken down very quickly by the liver, are also not effective if given enterally.

Because caffeine is not broken down by the acid in the stomach, it is readily absorbed by the blood vessels in the walls of the stomach and intestines. About one-sixth of a dose of caffeine is absorbed through the stomach walls, and most of the remainder is absorbed through the wall of the duodenum, the first section of the small intestine. In addition, caffeine is metabolized relatively slowly by the liver. These properties make it a suitable drug for enteral administration.

The speed with which caffeine gets from the mouth into the bloodstream depends on a number of factors. Absorption is slower, for example, when the stomach is full or after prolonged fasting. Usually a single dose of caffeine passes into the bloodstream within 30 minutes of administration.

Distribution and Doses

Blood containing caffeine flows from the gastrointestinal tract to the liver and then to the heart, from where it is circulated quickly throughout the body, including through the brain. The process whereby a drug spreads throughout the body is known as *distribution*. Caffeine is distributed to all of the body's water—approximately 42 liters, or 60% of total body

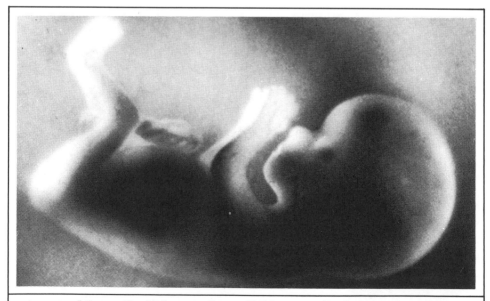

A normal 3-month-old human fetus. Children can be born with a caffeine dependency if their mothers continue to ingest the drug while pregnant.

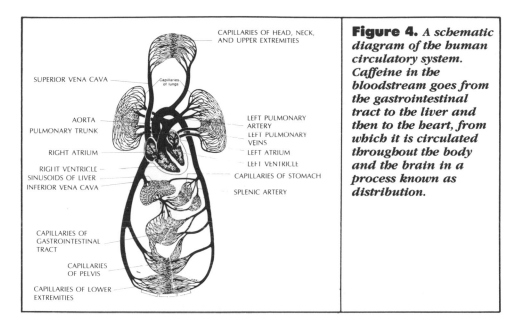

Figure 4. *A schematic diagram of the human circulatory system. Caffeine in the bloodstream goes from the gastrointestinal tract to the liver and then to the heart, from which it is circulated throughout the body and the brain in a process known as distribution.*

weight, in an adult male. Of this 42 liters of water, only 6 liters is in blood. Most of it—about 28 liters—is found in the cells of the body that make up the brain, muscles, and other tissues and the remainder is found between the cells. Because, unlike some drugs, caffeine is relatively insoluble in fat, it does not accumulate in body fat, a substance in which it could be stored for long periods.

The effect of a given amount of drug is directly related to the weight of the person or animal receiving the drug. This is because a heavier body will generally contain more water and therefore dilute a given drug dose more. The result is a lower drug concentration in the blood reaching the brain and the other organs where the drug has its effects. It is the drug's concentration in the blood that generally determines how strong an effect will be.

The relationship between dose, body weight, and drug concentration in the blood is clarified further in Table 7. One must note that the caffeine-concentration levels would occur only if all of the caffeine dose were distributed evenly throughout the body's water *before* any of the drug had been metabolized by the liver. Usually concentration levels would be higher because uneven distribution causes more caffeine to be in the blood than in other body fluids.

Table 7

Body Weight and Dose and Blood Concentration of Caffeine		
BODY WEIGHT	154 lbs	184.8 lbs
Amount of caffeine administered (mg)	105.00	105.00
Effective caffeine dose (mg/kg)	1.50	1.25
Caffeine concentration in blood (mg/l)	2.50	2.10

Metabolism

Each time caffeine-containing blood passes through the liver, a small portion of the caffeine is metabolized. The caffeine removed from the blood is replaced by more of the drug returning from the body's other fluids. This process continues until eventually all of the caffeine has been metabolized by the liver.

The metabolism of caffeine is a complex process involving more than a dozen known metabolites, or products (see Chapter 4). Details of the process have become clear only in recent years, brought on by the advent of powerful equipment for distinguishing closely related chemicals and by the development of sophisticated techniques for labeling parts of the caffeine molecule and tracing their fate in the body.

The main metabolite of caffeine metabolism is 1,5-dimethylxanthine, known as paraxanthine. During later passes through the liver the paraxanthine is metabolized, producing, among other chemicals, 1-methylxanthine, which is the main metabolite of caffeine excreted in urine.

The strength of caffeine's effect on the body depends largely on the concentration of the drug in the blood circulating through the brain. This concentration reaches a peak between 30 and 60 minutes after caffeine is taken by mouth, after most of the caffeine has been absorbed from the gastrointestinal tract, and before much of it is metabolized by the liver. (Caffeine's direct action on the brain is discussed in Chapter 7.)

Caffeine continues to have an effect as long as it remains in the blood. The critical factor is the metabolizing activity of substances in the liver known as enzymes. A lower rate of metabolism means the drug remains in the body and produces its effects longer. The half-life of caffeine—the amount of time it takes for the liver to remove half of the amount that has been ingested—varies considerably from individual to individual. The usual adult half-life ranges from 2.5 to 10 hours, averaging about 4 hours. Most of the drug is removed from the body within 12 hours. Men and women tend to have similar average rates of caffeine metabolism, as do people of all ages. Because of the liver's role in caffeine metabolism, most kinds of liver disease, particularly liver disease related to alcohol abuse, increase caffeine half-life.

Use of other drugs can dramatically affect the rate of caffeine metabolism. On an average, smokers, whose caffeine half-life is approximately 3 hours, metabolize caffeine 50% faster than nonsmokers. Thus, smokers experience the effect of a given cup of coffee for a shorter period of time than do nonsmokers. In addition, caffeine and nicotine have opposite effects on the neurotransmitter adenosine (see Chapter 4). Perhaps smokers tend to drink more coffee than nonsmokers in order to compensate for these effects.

Some drugs reduce the rate of caffeine metabolism. Alcohol has this effect, as does cimetidine, which is used to treat stomach ulcers. Use of oral contraceptives can more than triple the half-life of caffeine. Thus, women taking the birth control pill tend to react strongly to a second caffeine

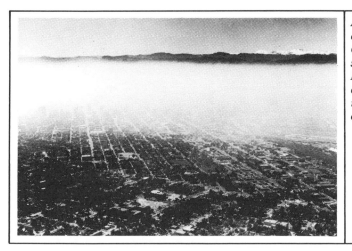

A blanket of smog covers Denver, Colorado. Pollution such as this contains PCBs, toxic chemicals that increase the rate of caffeine metabolism.

dose because residual caffeine from the earlier dose remains in the blood. Exposure to PCBs (polychlorinated biphenyls), considered to be major pollutants, also increases the rate of caffeine metabolism.

Some of the variability in rates of caffeine metabolism is inherited. Asians, for example, appear to metabolize caffeine differently and more slowly than Caucasians. Some of the variability, however, may be the result of experience with caffeine. Regular caffeine users may metabolize caffeine more quickly, though this has not yet been proven.

The rate of caffeine metabolism declines during pregnancy, particularly during the last few weeks. It returns to normal levels in the mother a few days after giving birth.

North American women tend to reduce their caffeine intake as pregnancy progresses. British women, whose caffeine intake is mainly from tea, do not reduce their caffeine consumption as much. Because caffeine metabolism is slowed, the amount of caffeine circulating in blood reaches high levels in many British pregnant women. Thus, the babies they are carrying receive high doses of caffeine. Why these differences in caffeine use occur is not known.

Most of the enzymes that metabolize caffeine are not present in the livers of newborn babies. Caffeine in their blood has to be excreted through the urine, which is a slow process—the half-life of caffeine in newborn babies is ap-

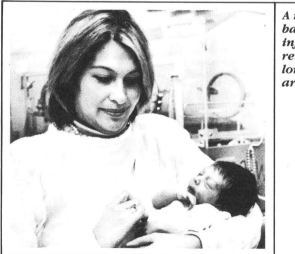

A mother holds her newborn baby. Caffeine received by infants before birth can remain in their system for as long as 85 hours after they are born.

proximately 85 hours. As the enzymes begin to be produced, the half-life decreases. By 2 months of age the half-life is close to 27 hours, and by 4 months it is 14 hours. At 6 months the infant's caffeine half-life averages between 2 and 3 hours— below the adult level. It remains below the adult level until adolescence.

Paradoxically, the livers of newborns convert theophylline into caffeine more efficiently than do adult livers (see Chapter 4). As much as 75% of a dose of theophylline given to a newborn may be converted to caffeine, as compared to 6% for adults. Theophylline is used in the treatment of breathing problems in newborn babies, especially premature babies. The effectiveness of theophylline in treating breathing difficulties may depend on this conversion. In fact, some researchers have suggested that breathing problems in newborn babies may occur because the babies are no longer getting the caffeine they were used to receiving from their caffeine-consuming mothers. When a baby is breast-fed, it continues to ingest caffeine and thus avoids caffeine withdrawal. This is because the milk of a caffeine-using woman has a caffeine concentration of about 50% that of the mother's blood.

As well as being secreted into milk, caffeine is also secreted from blood into saliva and semen. Compared with the concentration in the user's blood, the concentration in his or her saliva is about 75%, and that in semen is about 100%, or approximately equal to the level in the blood.

Elimination

Except in newborn babies, there is very little *elimination* of unchanged caffeine. Only small amounts of unmetabolized caffeine are eliminated in feces and in body fluids other than urine, and less than 3% of the ingested caffeine appears unchanged in urine. Most of the caffeine is excreted into the urine in the form of caffeine metabolites. This is done by the kidneys as the blood flows through them (see Figure 4) at a rate dependent on the amount of urine produced. Even though only a small amount of ingested caffeine appears in urine, the average concentration of caffeine found in urine is relatively high—about 40% higher than in blood—because the actual volume of urine is small compared with that of blood.

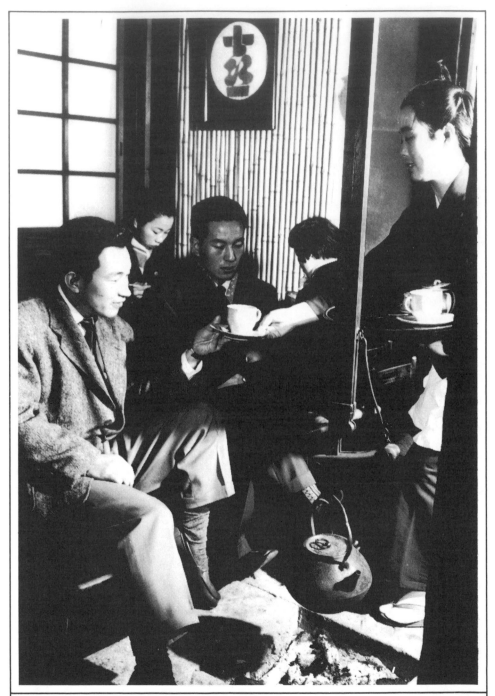

Customers are served in a Tokyo coffee shop as they warm their feet by the fire. In many parts of the world the partaking of coffee and tea is a ritualistic, often communal, event.

CHAPTER 6

VARIATION IN RESPONSE TO CAFFEINE

When people talk about the acute effects of caffeine, or those of any other drug, they usually focus on the desirable effects—at least when reference is being made to moderate doses. The acute effects of large amounts of a drug, however, are generally toxic and sometimes fatal. Mention of the chronic effects of a drug usually, but not always, refers to the undesirable effects.

Caffeine is used at least partly because of the short-term positive effects it is believed to cause in mood and behavior. An understanding of what these effects are, and whether they even exist, may help one better understand why the use of caffeine-containing beverages has such an important place in human behavior.

Knowledge of a drug's acute effects can lead to a more complete understanding of what causes the undesirable chronic effects. The chronic effects of a drug, including its contribution to certain diseases, is often the result of the body's repeated experience of the drug's acute effects. If one could show, for example, that every dose of caffeine has an effect on the heart, it could be determined whether caffeine use actually causes the heart disease with which it sometimes appears to be associated.

Why do some individuals appear to be more strongly affected by a given dose of the drug than others? Some people report that even a single cup of coffee in the evening disturbs their sleep. Others claim that before retiring they can drink several cups and experience few or no effects. A number of factors explain this wide variation.

Tolerance

The most important factor contributing to individual variation in the acute effects of caffeine is *tolerance*, a condition that occurs with prolonged use of almost all drugs. Tolerance to a particular effect of a drug has occurred when the same dose of a drug no longer produces the effect it did initially. Thus, in order to achieve the original effect the dose must be increased.

Because repeated administration of a drug can reduce its acute effects, and even mask them entirely, studies of acute effects must use experimental subjects with no previous experience with caffeine—unless, of course, the study intends to focus on the acute effects of caffeine on tolerant subjects.

The observation that heavy users of caffeine require more of the drug to get them going in the morning is not necessarily evidence of tolerance to caffeine. These heavy users may have always been relatively insensitive to caffeine's effects. Tolerance is *acquired* insensitivity. Evidence for it can only come from observations of changes in the effects of caffeine with repeated use.

An example of tolerance to caffeine comes from a study of blood pressure in three groups of healthy adults. Reported in the medical literature in 1981, it remains one of the few studies of caffeine's effects in which factors affecting the development of tolerance were properly controlled. Group A (9 subjects) was given 250 mg of caffeine in a strong-tasting drink after they had abstained from caffeine for 24 days.

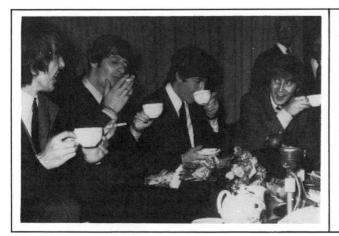

The Beatles at a press conference. Smokers metabolize caffeine much more quickly than do nonsmokers— in heavy smokers the rate can be up to twice as fast. Recent studies show that concentrations of caffeine in the blood rise sharply in those who quit smoking but continue to drink the same amount of coffee.

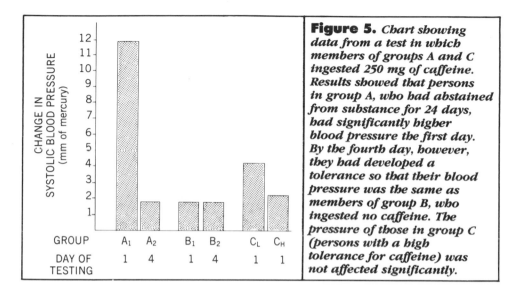

Figure 5. *Chart showing data from a test in which members of groups A and C ingested 250 mg of caffeine. Results showed that persons in group A, who had abstained from substance for 24 days, had significantly higher blood pressure the first day. By the fourth day, however, they had developed a tolerance so that their blood pressure was the same as members of group B, who ingested no caffeine. The pressure of those in group C (persons with a high tolerance for caffeine) was not affected significantly.*

Group B (9 subjects) abstained from caffeine for 24 days but received no caffeine in their strong-tasting drink. Group C (16 subjects) also received 250 mg of caffeine in the strong-tasting drink, but they had continued to drink their regular three cups of coffee a day until 24 hours before the test.

All subjects received the strong-tasting drink three times a day for 6 days, and every day each subject's blood pressure was measured both before and two hours after the 9 A.M. administration of the drink.

The data indicate that in every subject, regardless of history or caffeine dosage, average blood pressure was higher after consuming the strong-tasting drink (see Figure 5). Clearly, something other than caffeine must have caused the increase. Perhaps each subject's blood pressure was normally higher at 11:00 A.M. than at 9:00 A.M. Whatever the reason, the changes in blood pressure in the subjects who received caffeine (those in Groups A and C) needed to be compared with this baseline increase.

That Bar A_1 is very much higher than Bar B_1 indicates that caffeine, ingested after 24 days of abstinence, initially produces a significant increase in blood pressure. However, on the fourth day of caffeine administration there was no difference between these two groups, indicating that complete tolerance to the effect of caffeine on blood pressure had developed in the subjects in Group A.

In analyzing the results, Group C was split into two sub-groups according to how much caffeine was found in the subject's blood just prior to receiving the strong-tasting, caffeine-containing drink. Sub-group C_L had less than 1 mg of caffeine per liter of blood, indicating that these subjects usually drank weak coffee and/or that they metabolized caffeine quickly. As shown in Figure 5, the caffeine significantly increased the blood pressure of these subjects, though the increase was considerably less than that for the subjects in Group A, who had abstained from caffeine for 24 days rather than for 1 day.

Subjects in Sub-group C_H had more than 1 mg of caffeine per liter of blood when originally tested, indicating that they usually drank stronger coffee and/or metabolized caffeine slowly. Their blood pressure increased insignificantly after they consumed caffeine in the strong-tasting drink.

Three conclusions can be drawn from this study:

1. A single 250-mg dose of caffeine can produce a significant increase in blood pressure in abstinent subjects.

2. Within four days, repeated administration of caffeine produces significant tolerance to the effect of the drug on blood pressure.

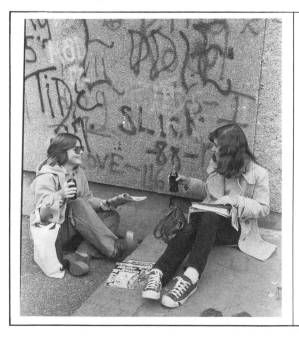

Teenagers in New York City enjoy Cokes during a break from school. Most of the caffeine consumed in the United States comes from cola beverages, but few who drink them are aware that they are also ingesting a powerful drug.

OMNI-PHOTO COMMUNICATIONS, INC./© ERIC KROLL

3. In some subjects, tolerance to caffeine's effect on blood pressure persists even after 24 hours of abstinence. In other subjects, one day's abstinence does reduce though does not entirely eliminate tolerance to these effects.

In this same study, the researchers also found evidence of tolerance to caffeine's acute effects on the rate of breathing and on the amounts of certain chemicals in the blood and urine. Other studies have shown, with differing degrees of statistical significance, that tolerance can occur to caffeine's effects on urine and saliva production, on sleep, and, in animals, on general movement and on the activity of nerve cells in certain parts of the brain.

Because there have been few properly conducted studies of tolerance to caffeine, knowledge of caffeine's acute effects is uncertain. Many findings that caffeine has no effect on a particular function of the body may have occurred because the experimenters were using subjects who were tolerant to that effect.

Other Sources of Variation

Even after differences in tolerance, rate of metabolism, rate of absorption, and body weight are allowed for, there may still be causes of variation in response to caffeine. One additional source of variation may be found in the nervous system. For example, there may be inherited differences in the structure of the gaps between nerve cells that allow caffeine to compete more successfully for adenosine receptors in some individuals than in others. Such differences in the nervous system could explain the variations in response to caffeine with respect to personality that have been reported by some investigators (see Chapter 7).

Researchers who have compared children who use little caffeine (less than 50 mg/day) with children who use a lot (more than 500 mg/day) have suggested that the lower reactivity of the heavy users may be the result of exposure to maternal caffeine before birth.

The many possible sources of variation in individual responses to caffeine should always be considered when caffeine's effects are being discussed and investigated. The following chapters, which deal with caffeine's short-term effects, include much evidence that is contradictory, and this is probably because researchers have not paid careful enough attention to these sources of variation, particularly tolerance.

12:45 a.m.

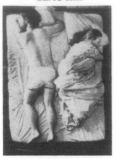

1:45 a.m.

2:45 a.m.

3 a.m.

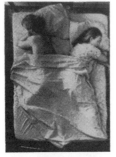

3:30 a.m.

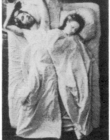

4:15 a.m.

5 a.m.

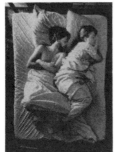

5:15 a.m.

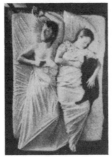

5:30 a.m.

5:45 a.m.

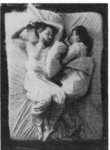

6 a.m.

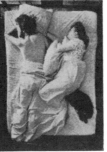

6:15 a.m.

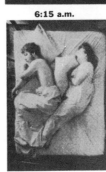

This series illustrates restless tossing and turning during the course of a night's sleep, a common complaint among caffeine users.

CHAPTER 7

CAFFEINE'S EFFECT ON THE BRAIN, BEHAVIOR, MOOD, AND SLEEP

*I*n textbooks of pharmacology—the branch of science that deals with the effects of drugs—caffeine is classified as a central nervous system stimulant. It is also known as an *analeptic drug*, or a substance that can restore strength, awaken, and invigorate. This chapter is concerned with the various properties that give caffeine its reputation as a stimulant or analeptic drug.

There is little concrete knowledge about caffeine's effects on the brain, behavior, and mood at normal doses—i.e., between 40 mg and 300 mg. Thus, much of this chapter, which mostly focuses on the effects of doses within this range, consists of qualified statements and contradictions. While at times this may seem confusing, it reflects the state of caffeine research, a problem with which researchers too must contend.

Brain

Statements that caffeine stimulates the central nervous system—the brain and the spinal cord—are based on very little actual observation of the central nervous system itself. Mention of caffeine stimulation usually refers to the drug's stimulation of behavior or mood. The assumption is that a certain degree of heightened brain activity is also involved.

Studies of changes in brain activity show that caffeine does have arousing effects. One way to measure this is to attach electrodes to a person's skull and record the patterns of electrical activity of his or her brain. It has been shown that the caffeine in a few cups of coffee causes the patterns to change from those typical of a resting, awake person to those typical of an alert and active person. Careful observations of the brains of animals have shown that caffeine enhances the activity of cells both at the surface of the cortex (that area of the brain associated with complex sensations and behavior), and in the deeper structures of the brain (those areas associated with primitive behavior and emotion).

As discussed in Chapter 4, the current theory is that caffeine interferes with the actions of the neurotransmitter adenosine. Though evidence in support of this theory is accumulating, because of the brain's complexity we are still a long way from explaining every feature of caffeine's actions on the central nervous system.

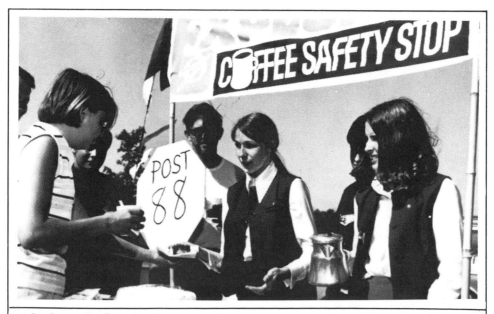

A highway "safety shop" serves coffee to weary travelers. Although caffeine does combat fatigue and increase alertness, it cannot "sober up" an intoxicated driver. An individual's motor functions remain just as impaired from alcohol after he or she drinks coffee as they were before.

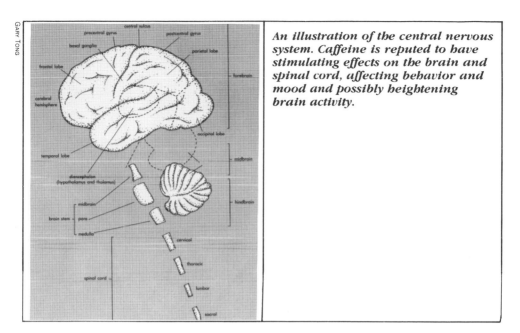

GARY TONG

An illustration of the central nervous system. Caffeine is reputed to have stimulating effects on the brain and spinal cord, affecting behavior and mood and possibly heightening brain activity.

Behavior

Apart from the effect on sleep (see below), the clearest effect of 150 mg of caffeine—equivalent to two average cups of coffee, or about three cans of Coke—is an increase in general bodily movement. This has mostly been observed in animals, although when the right measurements are made this effect can also be seen in humans. However, even this most obvious of behavioral effects is sometimes not found. In fact, when investigators gave these relatively low doses of caffeine to experimental animals, occasionally *reductions* in general activity were observed. Almost all studies have found that animals receiving very high doses of caffeine (six cups or more of coffee) show reduced general activity.

In humans, studies of caffeine's effects on activity have focused on work output and athletic performance. The usual finding is that the caffeine in several average cups of coffee prolongs the amount of time an individual can perform physically exhausting work. The quality of the physical work is *not* improved, except when the performance only depends on endurance, as in long-distance running, cross-country skiing, and cycling. This effect on performance seems greater if the work load is constant rather than increasing, if the work is being done at a high altitude rather than at sea level, and at normal rather than at cold temperatures. Caffeine has also been shown to shorten the time needed to recover from exhausting work.

In Tibet, an area averaging between 12,000 feet and 17,000 feet above sea level, tea has been used for centuries as an aid to endurance. According to William Emboden, the author of *Narcotic Plants*,

> *Weary horses and mules are given large vessels of tea to increase their capacity to work. Mules are said to be gamboling like colts as a result of their tea rations.... The distance between villages is accounted for in terms of the number of cups of tea necessary to sustain the person traveling that route. It has been ascertained that three cups of tea is equal to eight kilometers.*

How caffeine might enhance endurance is not understood. However, we know that the avoidance of exhaustion must involve a slowing down in the rate at which glycogen— a muscle's source of energy—is used up. Caffeine must either

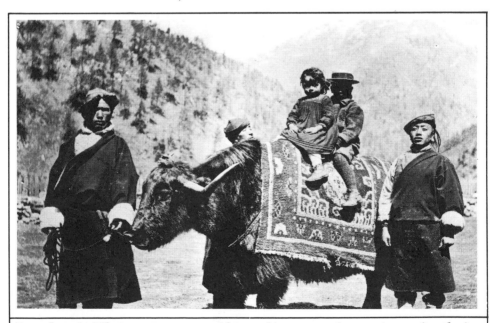

Travelers in Tibet use tea as an aid to endurance and as a measuring device: the distance between two places is gauged by the amount of tea needed to sustain the people during the trek.

cause more efficient use of glycogen or facilitate greater use of energy sources external to muscles, such as body fat and blood sugars. Preliminary research in this area suggests that caffeine acts both ways. Caffeine's effect on the body's use of energy is discussed further in the next chapter.

Some studies have found little or no significant enhancement of endurance by caffeine. Even a very small improvement, however, could make an important difference in athletic competition. An improvement by 0.6% in the time taken to run 10,000 meters might not be scientifically significant, but it would have reduced Alberto Cova's winning time at the 1984 Olympic Games in Los Angeles (actually 27.79 minutes) by enough for him to have broken the record of 27.64 minutes set by Lasse Viren at the 1972 games in Munich.

Athletes have, in fact, used caffeine to enhance their performance. Indeed, in 1962 caffeine was classified as a "doping agent" by the International Olympic Committee. It was removed from the list in 1972, but put back for the 1984 games; caffeine remained on the list for the 1988 games. A

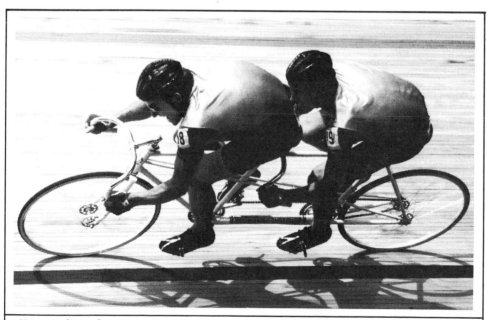

Two cyclists during a race. Because of caffeine's stimulating effects, the Olympic Committee declared the drug a "doping agent" in 1962 and again in 1984; an excessive dose of caffeine disqualified an athlete.

1982 study of 775 Belgian racing cyclists of many ages and levels of performance found that while their *average* regular caffeine use was lower than that of the general population, some professional cyclists were probably using excessive amounts of caffeine to help them in their races. The authors of this study suggested that caffeine levels in the urine in excess of 15 micrograms per milliliter should be considered evidence of caffeine doping. These levels could be achieved if an athlete drank three or four cups of strong coffee just before an event. As of 1991 the Olympic Committee has continued to place caffeine on its list of doping agents: athletes may not compete if they have in excess of 12 micrograms of caffeine per milliliter of urine, an amount, the Committee says, that can show up in tests conducted within 2–3 hours of drinking 6–8 cups of coffee.

Where hand steadiness or fine motor coordination is required, rather than simple endurance, caffeine can cause a worsening of performance. For example, consumption of two or three cups of coffee has been found to reduce skill at needle threading and handwriting. Not all studies have found a negative effect of caffeine on this kind of behavior, however. Some have actually shown an improvement. The question of whether caffeine has a consistent effect on skilled behavior is still to be answered.

Caffeine disruption of fine motor coordination is exhib-

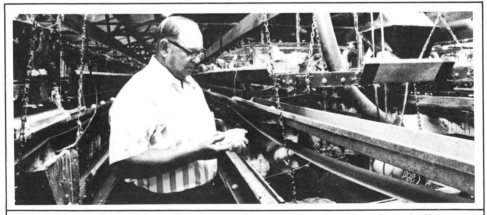

Some studies show that caffeine can improve performance of unchallenging, simple tasks such as egg inspection, which are highly repetitive and require long attention spans.

ited as an increase in hand or arm tremors, sometimes called the "coffee shakes." Recent work, using equipment capable of detecting small, often invisible, movements, has confirmed the relationship between these effects and caffeine. At lower doses (150 mg) the drug may act only to enhance tremors already present and unrelated to caffeine use.

Perhaps the most interesting question about caffeine is whether it has an effect on intellectual activity. Advertisers have promoted coffee as "The Think Drink," but the evidence as to whether caffeine helps one think better is even more confusing than the evidence supporting caffeine's relationship to skilled behavior.

One researcher has suggested that the following three effects are produced by moderate doses of caffeine (150 mg–300 mg, equivalent to 3–6 cans of Coke):

1. Caffeine improves performance of simple tasks that require attention rather than memory. Examples of such tasks are searching for particular two-letter sequences in long strings of letters; watching out for defective items passing on a conveyor belt; and reacting quickly to a signal. In this case caffeine seems to delay deterioration in performance due to boredom or fatigue.

2. Caffeine worsens performance that involves short-term memory, such as searching for particular six-letter sequences in long strings of letters, or reciting lists of recently learned words. Caffeine may speed up the performance of these tasks, but more errors are made.

3. Caffeine affects performance of complex tasks in ways that depend on the personality of the user. Impulsivity is an important feature of personality. Impulsive people tend to sacrifice accuracy for speed and also tend to be more aroused in the evening than in the morning. When caffeine is given in the morning to people rated as highly impulsive by personality tests, it improves their performance at complex tasks such as proofreading for grammatical and typographical errors. When caffeine is ingested in the evening when these people are more aroused, it has the opposite effect. People who achieve low scores when being measured for impulsivity are affected in the opposite way. Their performance at complex intellectual tasks is worsened in the morning, when their arousal is high, and improved in the evening, when their arousal is low.

The reliability of some of these findings, however, is questionable. Contrary data on each of these points have been reported in the scientific literature. Moreover, people cannot be categorized as impulsive or non-impulsive with a great deal of precision. And even if this characteristic could be reliably and accurately measured, most people fall somewhere in the middle. Thus their performance of complex intellectual tasks is neither worsened nor improved by caffeine, whether in the morning or in the evening.

The possible relationship between personality type and an individual's sensitivity to, metabolism of, and tolerance to caffeine makes research in this area very difficult—so many complicating factors have to be taken into account.

The effects of caffeine on behavior may also depend on whether or not subjects know they have taken caffeine. One study found that caffeine improved performance of a task only when subjects knew they had ingested caffeine. In another study, subjects were given either capsules containing caffeine or a placebo. (A placebo is a substance that the subject cannot distinguish from the drug being tested and that has no detectable effect on the body.) Ninety minutes after ingesting the capsule, subjects could readily determine if they had been given the caffeine or a placebo. Researchers have to be very careful to take their subjects' knowledge of what is going on into account. Few do, and that is possibly why the research on the effects of caffeine on intellectual activity has been mostly inconclusive.

A question often asked about caffeine is whether it can counteract the adverse effects of drugs such as alcohol. In general, research in this area has also been inconclusive. With regards to caffeine and alcohol, both *synergistic effects* (when two drugs taken together produce effects greater than either drug alone) and *antagonistic effects* (when one drug counteracts the effects of another drug) have been observed.

In one recent study of reaction time, caffeine taken alone had no effect, alcohol increased reaction time (slowed the subject's response), and the caffeine/alcohol combination increased the reaction time even more. In another study, caffeine was found to counteract the negative effect of alcohol on the performance of mental arithmetic in male but not in female subjects. And a third study found that at low doses neither alcohol, nor caffeine, nor their combination had a measurable effect on skills involved in automobile driving, though the subjects reported feeling impaired after taking alcohol and more alert after ingesting caffeine.

Overall, the scientific evidence does not support the idea that a few cups of coffee will make a person fit to drive after three or four beers. In fact, the caffeine can make the driver of an automobile more dangerous. By heightening alertness, it may make drivers *believe* they can do things that in fact they are not capable of doing. Instead of being sleepy drunks, they become wide-awake and even more dangerous drunks.

Similarly, caffeine does not counteract the effects of phenobarbital and other barbiturates. Recent studies have shown, however, that caffeine appears to counteract the impairment of cognitive activity—that is, thinking caused by diazepam, the chemical that is the major ingredient in Valium and other tranquilizers.

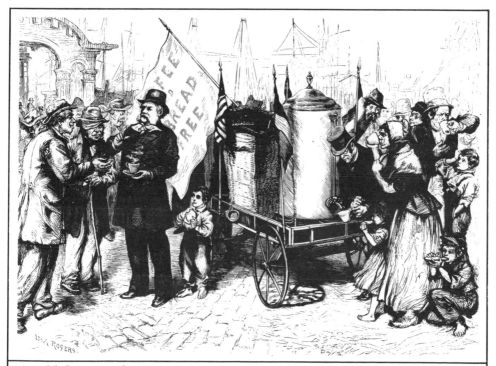

An old drawing shows temperance workers attempting to sober up the masses by serving them cups of hot coffee. Although caffeine is classified as a stimulant, it is not effective in counteracting the intoxicating effects of alcohol and barbiturates.

Mood

Another claim made in advertisements, probably referring to caffeine's effects on mood, is that "coffee calms you down— and picks you up." Research into caffeine's effects on mood has mostly involved psychiatric patients (see Chapter 10), though there have been a few studies on the general population. The results of these tests have been contradictory. Use of moderate to large amounts of caffeine (300 mg caffeine or more) has generally been found to produce feelings of tension and anxiety, but not always. Enhanced alertness has often been reported, along with greater vigor and reduced fatigue, but again not always. Other mood effects also seem inconsistent: for example, depression and anger have been found to be both increased and reduced by caffeine.

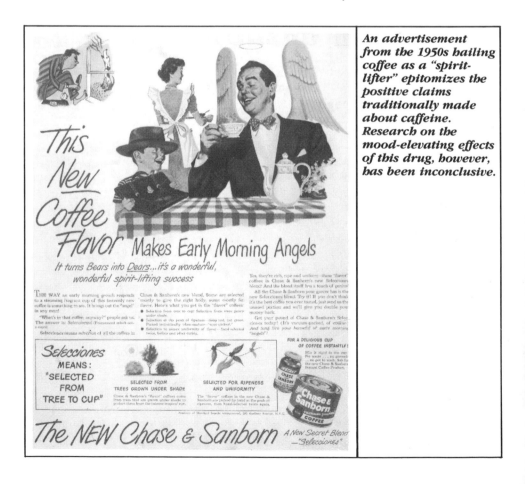

An advertisement from the 1950s hailing coffee as a "spirit-lifter" epitomizes the positive claims traditionally made about caffeine. Research on the mood-elevating effects of this drug, however, has been inconclusive.

These conflicting results may have occurred because the researchers did not take the regular caffeine use of their subjects into account. In one study in which proper account was taken, the researchers found that coffee drinkers experienced increased vigor and reduced fatigue, while noncoffee drinkers reported tension and anxiety. Another study involved children whose normal daily caffeine consumption was either less than 50 mg or more than 500 mg. The low consumers were more emotional and restless when they received about 200 mg caffeine. The high consumers were unaffected by the caffeine they received, but anxious when they ingested a placebo. These children were probably dependent on caffeine (see Chapter 10).

Are the mood changes that follow caffeine use related to performance? Does caffeine make people work better because it makes them feel more alert, or do they feel more alert because they are working better? Again, the evidence is contradictory.

As with performance, caffeine's effects on mood can depend strongly on whether or not the subjects know they are ingesting caffeine. One study found that just being told that caffeine was being given enhanced both the feeling of increased vigor and the feeling of reduced fatigue.

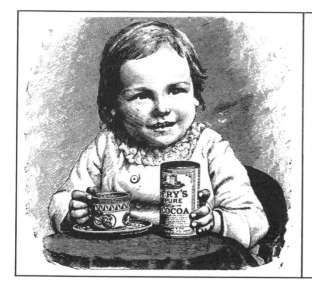

A young child enjoys a cup of cocoa, a beverage containing a low amount (about 2 mg per cup) of caffeine. Children whose daily caffeine intake is more than 500 mg are both calmed and invigorated by the drug, but may also become dependent on it.

Sleep

In contrast to what can be said about most of caffeine's effects on behavior and mood, it is possible to say with some certainty that the caffeine in a strong cup of coffee consumed an hour before going to bed will have some effect on the sleep of most people. The noticeable effects are an increase in the time it takes to fall asleep and a reduction in total sleep time.

In a recent Japanese study, after ingesting 150 mg of caffeine, 8 subjects took an average of 126 minutes to get to sleep, compared with 29 minutes for those who had not consumed caffeine. The caffeine users slept for a total of 281 minutes, compared with 444 minutes for the noncaffeine users. Recordings of the electrical activity of the brain during

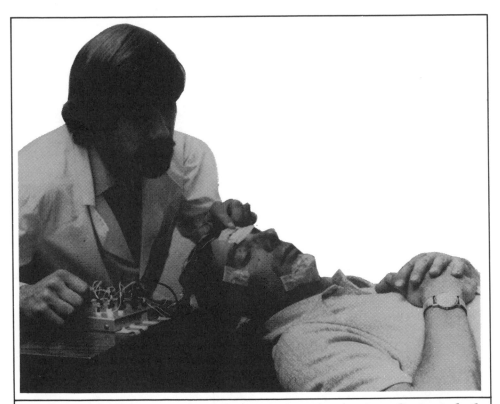

A scientist attaches electrodes to the head of a volunteer in order to study the effects of caffeine on sleeping patterns.

sleep showed that the caffeine consistently altered the normal sleep patterns. These findings are similar to those of many other studies, although studies using non-Asian subects usually produces less dramatic results.

Caffeine users are more readily aroused by sudden noises and exhibit an increase in body movements during sleep and a decrease in the reported quality of sleep. There is disagreement as to caffeine's effect on the phase of sleep known as REM, or rapid-eye-movement, sleep. Research has shown that it is during this phase, characterized by a specific type of electrical activity in the brain, that dreaming occurs. When caffeine is used, REM sleep tends to occur earlier. However, studies have shown that caffeine does not decrease REM sleep as alcohol and barbiturates do.

Although there are considerable differences in reactions to caffeine, people who consume a lot of caffeine usually sleep for shorter periods than people who use less. Not surprisingly, heavy caffeine use has been associated with chronic insomnia.

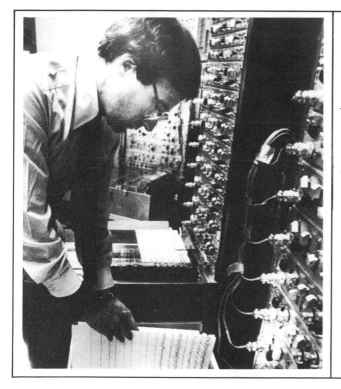

A researcher consults a chart depicting the influence of various drugs on the brain. Modern technology enables scientists to partially isolate bodily structures like the central nervous system in order to study the effects of a substance such as caffeine.

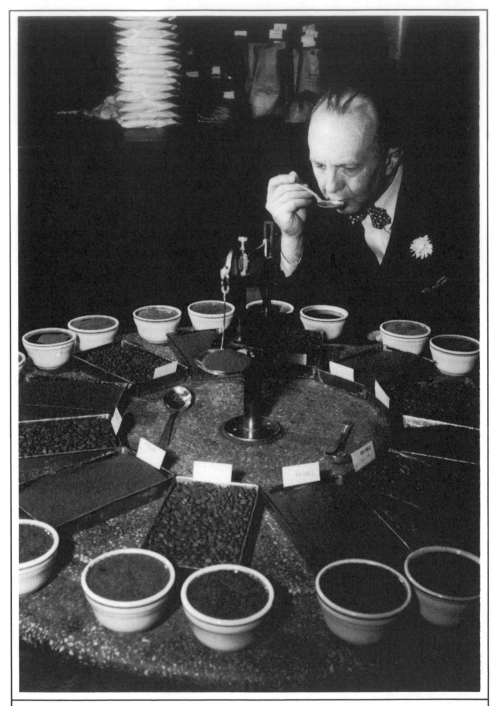

An inspector takes a sample from one of many cups of a coffee company's product. Taken in excess, caffeine can have toxic effects.

CHAPTER 8

THE ACUTE EFFECTS OF CAFFEINE

Caffeine reaches almost every part of the body and therefore has the potential to affect most of the body's functions. In fact, it does produce acute (short-term but often severe) effects on the cardiovascular system (the heart and blood vessels), on the digestive system, on breathing, on energy expenditure, and on urination. This property has also made it possible for caffeine to contribute to the therapeutic treatment of illnesses and diseases. But in addition, this characteristic enables caffeine to exhibit its toxic effects throughout the body. At the extreme, caffeine use can even be fatal.

As mentioned in the previous two chapters, scientists studying the effects of caffeine on the human body have not been particularly careful to take into consideration the large differences between individual responses. Because of this there remains considerable uncertainty about caffeine's effects.

Cardiovascular Effects

Two important measures of cardiovascular function are the pressure of the blood as it flows through the arteries (blood pressure) and the heart rate. Blood pressure is of special concern because high blood pressure is an indication of strain on the heart and blood vessels and of possible obstruction somewhere in the circulatory system. Anything that causes or adds to high blood pressure could be dangerous.

A person's blood pressure at any given time depends on two things: the output of blood from the heart and the resistance of the circulatory system to the flow of blood. The output from the heart is determined in part by the rate at which the heart beats. When both the resistance to blood flow and the volume of blood pumped through the system at each heart beat remain constant, blood pressure and heart rate rise and fall together.

Caffeine significantly increases the blood pressure in subjects who have been without the drug for some days (see Chapter 6). Complete tolerance to this effect develops quickly. In the study discussed in Chapter 6, this occurred after four days.

When the 1981 study was repeated using slightly hypertensive subjects—subjects whose blood pressure was a little higher than normal—similar results were found. However, some research has found a reduction in blood pressure as a result of caffeine administration, while other research has found none at all. Moreover, although the weight of evidence points to a transient (i.e., short-lived) increase in blood pressure as the main result of caffeine use, there are recent reports that people who consume heavy amounts of coffee, even when they are not under the influence of caffeine, tend to have slightly higher blood pressure than people who use little or no coffee.

Increased heart rate usually accompanies the use of caffeine, although the change is generally small and not statistically significant. In some studies, including the one mentioned above on slightly hypertensive subjects, reduced heart rate was found after caffeine administration. Other researchers have reported that caffeine causes an initial decrease and then an increase in heart rate.

Similar confusion exists concerning caffeine's effects on the circulatory system's resistance to blood flow. Some researchers have found dilation (widening) of blood vessels, particularly those in the brain. But both constriction of and a lack of any effect on blood vessels have also been observed.

A recent concern has been the possible role of caffeine in the occurrence of arrhythmias—irregularities in heart beat, sometimes known as palpitations. Forms of arrhythmias are thought to be involved in some cases of death from heart failure. A well-publicized experiment, reported in 1983, dem-

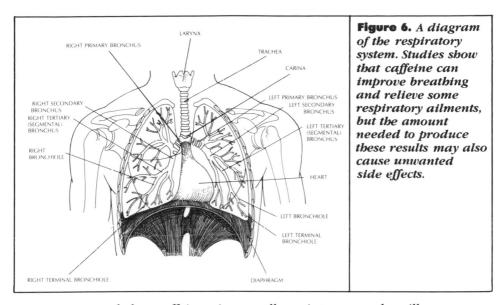

Figure 6. *A diagram of the respiratory system. Studies show that caffeine can improve breathing and relieve some respiratory ailments, but the amount needed to produce these results may also cause unwanted side effects.*

LARYNX

RIGHT PRIMARY BRONCHUS

TRACHEA

CARINA

RIGHT SECONDARY BRONCHUS

LEFT PRIMARY BRONCHUS
LEFT SECONDARY BRONCHUS

RIGHT TERTIARY (SEGMENTAL) BRONCHUS

LEFT TERTIARY (SEGMENTAL) BRONCHUS

RIGHT BRONCHIOLE

HEART

LEFT BRONCHIOLE

LEFT TERMINAL BRONCHIOLE

RIGHT TERMINAL BRONCHIOLE

DIAPHRAGM

onstrated that caffeine given orally or intravenously will reliably produce arrhythmias in subjects who had previous arrhythmic symptoms. However, a 1989 study, equally well-publicized, concluded that moderate doses of caffeine—the equivalent of 3 or 4 cups of coffee or 5–6 cans of Coke—do not pose a threat even to people with serious arrhythmias.

Respiratory Effects

Caffeine has been shown to increase the rate of breathing by heightening the sensitivity of the part of the brain that responds to the level of carbon dioxide in the blood. Caffeine can improve the depth of breathing by strengthening the action of the diaphragm, which is the major muscle involved with inhaling and exhaling (see Figure 6). One study has found that caffeine could be useful for people with lung disease who suffer from breathlessness.

Asthmatic patients have difficulty breathing because their bronchial passages become constricted. Theophylline (see Chapter 4) has long been used as a drug that dilates the bronchial passage and thus makes breathing easier for asthmatics. A recent comparison found that caffeine was also effective. However, the effective dose (the equivalent of about 9 average cups of coffee for an average-size person) produced unwanted side effects in most patients, notably shakiness and tremors.

Energy Expenditure and Weight Loss

Caffeine's short-term effects on the body's use of energy might be of interest to people who wish to lose weight. When ingested with a meal, caffeine increases the rate at which the food is converted into usable energy. When caffeine is taken between meals, it causes fats to be transferred from deposits in the cells to the bloodstream. Here, as *free fatty acids* they can be used as energy by most of the organs of the body.

Caffeine also raises the activity level of the body, which can mean that the energy derived from food is used up in exercise rather than being stored as fat. In addition, caffeine stimulates the temperature-regulating centers of the body, which in turn produces an increase in body temperature. To sustain this change, energy that might have otherwise been deposited as fat is used. Thus, even when the body is at rest a greater amount of food is burned.

Caffeine is a common ingredient in nonprescription diet aids, sometimes also known as appetite suppressants. However, there is no evidence that caffeine does indeed reduce appetite for food.

Despite the apparent relationship between caffeine's effects and weight loss, and though regular caffeine administration to animals has been shown to contribute to their losing weight, still it is not clear whether, in the long term, caffeine use contributes to weight loss in humans. Even if caffeine proved to be a weight-loss aid, one must consider this drug's other effects before advocating its use for this purpose. Frequently a drug's negative side effects make its use highly undesirable and dangerous. In addition, for a weight-loss program to be successful and lead to permanent weight loss, it must also include a change both in diet and life-style.

Digestion and Excretion

Drinking coffee increases the secretion of acid into the stomach, but it may be that, in addition to caffeine, other coffee components produce this effect. Although caffeine stimulates acid secretion, it also reduces the peristaltic action of the stomach, the action that causes the emptying of the stomach's contents into the small intestine. Caffeine also slows down the passage of material through the small intestine, yet speeds its passage through the large intestine.

All of the above-mentioned effects can contribute to digestive upset, and even to ulcers of the stomach and small intestine. People who already suffer from digestive upset are usually advised to give up caffeine-containing beverages. In fact, there is evidence that these people are more strongly affected by caffeine than are healthy people. One study, for example, found that in normal subjects 250 mg of caffeine raised the rate at which the stomach secreted hydrochloric acid from 200 mg per hour to 2,000 mg per hour. This effect disappeared within 90 minutes. In patients with ulcers in the small intestine, the same amount of caffeine raised the acid secretion rate from 300 mg per hour to 4,700 mg per hour. After two hours, the rate was still above 3,000 mg per hour.

As well as these effects on the digestive system, coffee and tea also reduce the body's absorption of specific nutrients, particularly iron, an essential mineral. The specific chemical or chemicals that cause the inhibition of iron uptake are not known, but caffeine and the tannins and other components of tea are the most likely agents. In addition to this, caffeine's ability to increase urination—by 30% for up to three hours following ingestion—can cause significant increases in the excretion in urine of calcium, magnesium, and sodium. Though some tolerance does develop to this effect, it could contribute to a deficiency in these minerals.

Caffeine as Medicine

Along with caffeine's beneficial effects on breathing, the drug is also successful in inducing breathing in newborn babies who experience breathing failure and continue to have spells of *apnea*, or cessation of breathing for more than 20 seconds.

Caffeine is frequently included in both prescription and nonprescription headache preparations and other pain relievers. The amount is small—much less per tablet than in an average cup of coffee. Exactly why caffeine was first included in these products along with analgesic drugs (pain relievers) such as aspirin and acetaminophen is not known, though it may have been added to counter possible depressant effects of these drugs. Caffeine may also have been included because it is especially effective as a remedy for headaches caused by caffeine withdrawal (see Chapter 10). But certainly few scientists and physicians originally assumed it was meant to increase the effectiveness of the painkillers.

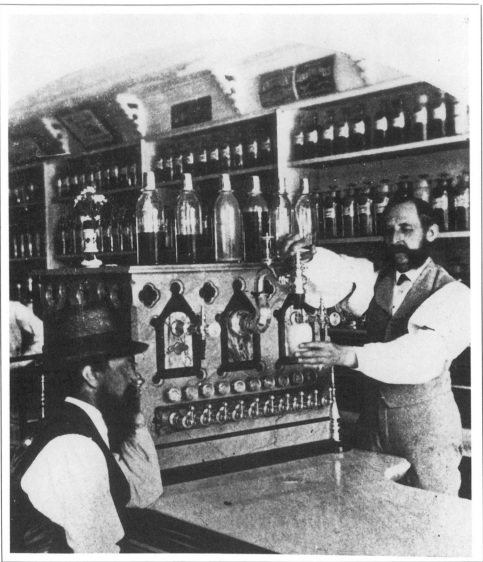

THE BETTMANN ARCHIVE

The drugstore soda fountain, a fixture of American life for more than half a century, owes its origins to Coca-Cola. The beverage was invented in 1886 by a Georgia pharmacist and sold in his store as a combination headache remedy and stimulant. Although the original formula contained wine and coca leaves, the wine had been replaced by caffeine in the form of kola nut extract by 1892, when the Coca-Cola Company was formed. Widespread distribution of this so-called health beverage to drugstores throughout the country soon followed.

In fact, in 1977 the U.S. Food and Drug Administration issued a report that stated that there was no evidence that caffeine helped analgesics relieve pain.

Since that time, however, research has shown that the addition of caffeine does indeed increase an analgesic's effectiveness and reduces the time needed for the drug to take effect. When combined with caffeine, 30% less analgesic is needed. This characteristic of caffeine is true not only for headache relief but also for a wide variety of pains, including those from oral surgery and childbirth. How caffeine enhances analgesia is not known.

Research has also suggested that caffeine may enhance the much more potent analgesic effects of the opiate drugs, including morphine and heroin. However, to date, physicians have used caffeine only as an antidote for opiate overdoses. Injections of caffeine into an opiate user's muscles counteract the effects of opiate poisoning on the brain, and restore the user's breathing if it has failed.

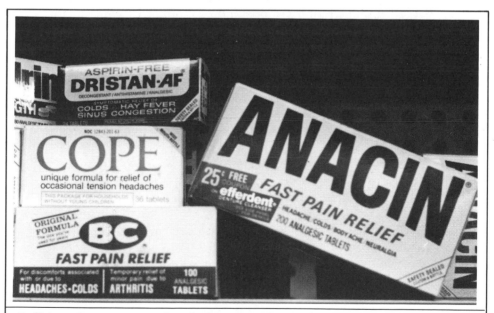

Caffeine alone can ease headaches; its role in other forms of pain relief is enhanced by combining it with analgesics such as aspirin and acetaminophen. In this form caffeine is widely available in numerous prescription and over-the-counter medicines.

Caffeine has also been used as an aid to fertility. A major cause of human infertility is sperm that are not mobile enough to reach and fertilize the egg. Studies of nonhuman mammals have shown that when caffeine is added to semen it can increase the mobility of their sperm and enhance fertilization. Studies of humans have produced similar findings regarding increased mobility, and at least one recent study suggests that, in fact, fertility too is enhanced by caffeine. According to the findings, women are twice as likely to become pregnant if prior to artificial insemination caffeine is added to the semen of their infertile mates. However, the concentration of caffeine used to achieve this effect is high—approximately 1,500 mg/liter, or more than three times the concentration of caffeine in the average cup of coffee (approximately 436 mg/liter). The possible negative side effects of such high concentrations of caffeine used in this way are not yet known.

Caffeine as a Poison

Death from a caffeine overdose has usually involved accidental administration by hospital personnel of caffeine by injection or by tablet, or suicide using caffeine-containing tablets. (One unusual case involved giving an enema of very strong coffee.) The lowest dose of caffeine known to have caused death in an adult is 3,200 mg, administered intravenously by a nurse who believed that the syringe contained another drug. Children have died from caffeine overdose after eating many wake-up, weight-control, or other caffeine-containing pills.

The acute fatal dose of caffeine taken by mouth is at least 5,000 mg—the equivalent of about 40 strong cups of coffee consumed in a very short period of time. Thus, death from a coffee "binge" is unlikely. Moreover, caffeine in high doses causes vomiting, which would add to the difficulty of consuming enough beverage to cause death.

The actual cause of death from caffeine poisoning is not known, though in general the toxic (poisonous) effects of a drug are related to the drug's effects at lower doses. A wide variety of effects have been observed in patients who have received about 1,000 mg of caffeine, including the following:

1. abnormally fast or deep breathing (hyperventilation)

2. rapid heart beat (tachycardia)
3. involuntary, uncoordinated muscle contractions (convulsions)
4. rapid, uncoordinated twitching of the heart (ventricular fibrillation)
5. low levels of potassium in blood (hypokalemia)
6. high levels of blood sugar and ketone bodies in urine, as in diabetes (glycosuria and ketonuria)

The prolongation of any of these effects of large doses of caffeine can lead to death. Some physicians have noted that caffeine poisoning resembles the condition that can occur when diabetics do not take insulin or when their insulin fails to regulate the fat and glucose levels in their blood. Among diabetics this condition is the most common cause of early death.

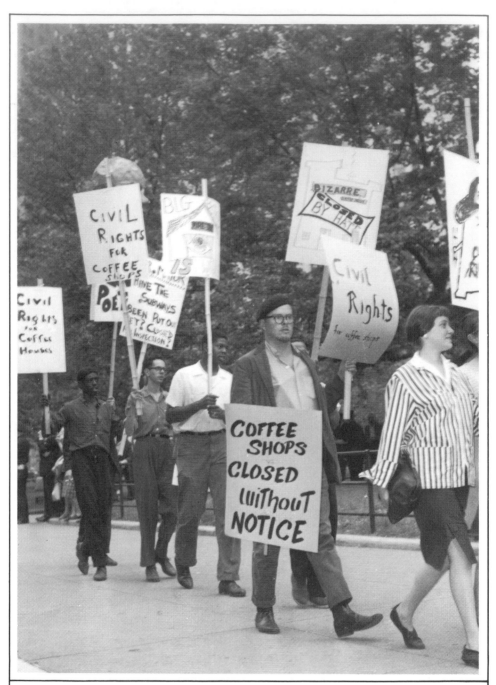

Members of the Beat Generation in New York City protest the closing of their favorite coffee houses. Drinking coffee was a communal pastime not only to the hippies of the 1960s but also to turn-of-the-century bohemians, who drank the beverage incessantly.

CHAPTER 9

DEPENDENCE ON CAFFEINE

A woman who regulary used more than 500 mg of caffeine per day was told to quit consuming this drug because it was causing irregularities in her heartbeat. She quit many times, but on each occasion, after about 18 hours she developed a head pain, initially "behind the eyes" and "in the back of the head." The pain spread throughout her head, peaking three hours after onset as a "splitting headache," accompanied by a mild runny nose, moderate fatigue, and persistent yawning. During the headache she could smell coffee even when none was present. Aspirin alone did not help, but headache pills that included 65 mg of caffeine per tablet provided some relief.

One day, in desperation, she rapidly consumed two strong cups of coffee, or at least 240 mg of caffeine. Her headache and other withdrawal symptoms disappeared within 90 minutes, but her irregular heartbeat returned. She found that if she did not take caffeine in one form or another the headache would persist for at least 36 hours.

A man who regularly used about 1,000 mg of caffeine per day volunteered to take part in a study during which he was required to go without caffeine for 72 hours or more a number of times over a period of 6 months. He reported various symptoms of caffeine withdrawal at regular intervals during each of the 72-hour periods. Usually a headache developed first, beginning at about 6 hours after quitting, followed by fatigue, a runny nose, leg pains, sweating, and then, at 16 hours, general muscle pains.

The symptoms increased in intensity throughout the 72-hour period. The headache and leg pains were the most severe, followed closely by the muscle pains, with the other symptoms having moderate severity.

At 72 hours the man was given decaffeinated coffee, sometimes with 115 mg of caffeine added. He did not know which he was being given. However, when he received caffeine the symptoms disappeared within 3 hours. Otherwise they continued.

These two case studies illustrate what is known as caffeine withdrawal, or the physical and psychological effects associated with the discontinuance of chronic caffeine use. The appearance of withdrawal symptoms is an indication that an individual has become physically dependent upon, or addicted to, a drug. Physical dependence, which may also include the tendency to increase drug dosage, is an adaptation of the body to the continued presence of a drug. Another type of dependence, psychological dependence, is a condi-

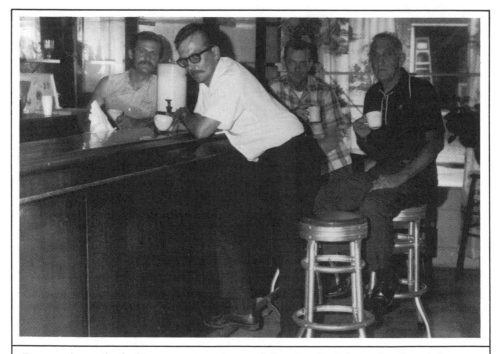

Recovering alcoholics recapture part of the ritual of their drinking days at a coffee bar that serves only nonalcoholic beverages.

tion in which the drug user craves a drug to maintain a sense of well-being and feels discomfort when deprived of it. Regular use of caffeine can produce both kinds of dependence.

Caffeine is capable of causing physical dependence in much the same way as other addictive drugs such as alcohol, heroin, nicotine, and the barbiturates. But unlike the symptoms associated with the opiates, caffeine withdrawal symptoms, though uncomfortable, are not life-threatening.

One characteristic symptom of caffeine withdrawal not mentioned in the two case studies is anxicty. As previously mentioned (see Chapter 7), feelings of tension and anxiety can be produced by *giving* subjects 300 mg or more of caffeine. These same feelings may also be the result of *withholding* caffeine from a regular user. Because the effects of giving a drug and the effects of withdrawing from it are usually *opposite* in nature, further examination may show that, though the same term is used, the anxiety caused by caffeine stimulation may be rather different from the anxiety of caffeine withdrawal.

Though some heavy users appear to be able to quit caffeine without distress, there is very little evidence to support this. In fact, most heavy users are aware of the link between quitting caffeine use and severe withdrawal headaches and know that these headaches can be relieved by ingesting caffeine. Therefore, it is quite difficult for them to quit.

The lowest level of daily consumption at which physical dependence occurs is approximately 350 mg per day—the equivalent of 4 average cups of coffee or 7 cans of Coke. It is likely that 20% or more of North Americans aged 15 years and over use at least this amount daily. Physical dependence on caffeine is thus a widespread phenomenon.

Physical dependence is not inherently harmful. It can become harmful, however, when drug administration is discontinued and/or when drug doses become so great and excessively ingested that they can cause illness and disease. If dependence can be sustained at doses that may not cause harm, the only problem with dependence is maintaining the supply of the drug so as to avoid the unpleasantness of withdrawal. Generally speaking, caffeine use is a threat to the health of normal adults only when regular consumption is in excess of about 600 mg per day. Because caffeine dependence occurs after a daily dose of 350 mg, persons using between

350 mg and 600 mg of caffeine per day can be dependent on the drug without apparent damage to their health.

Abstaining from caffeine, on the other hand, might very well pose a threat to the health of a dependent caffeine user. A person who uses a lot of caffeine and who skips his or her morning coffee usually experiences withdrawal symptoms, most apparently in the form of a headache. Such a person may be unusually irritable and thus accident-prone, socially disagreeable, and inclined to self-medication, none of which is consistent with good health.

Many of the reasons heavy caffeine users give for liking coffee may have as much to do with avoidance of withdrawal symptoms as with coffee's virtues. A recent study found that coffee drinkers say the following things about their preferred beverage, in order of emphasis:

1. It gives you a feeling of well-being.
2. It calms your nerves and makes you relax.
3. It helps you think and helps orient you.
4. It makes you less irritable.
5. It wakes you up and gets you going.
6. It reduces or avoids headache.
7. You would feel bad without it.
8. It stimulates you and gives you energy.

Caffeine is used to help newborn babies that experience apnea, or breathing difficulties (see Chapter 8). It is possible that some of these difficulties may be the result of caffeine withdrawal. Because their mothers used caffeine throughout pregnancy, at birth many babies will have already been exposed to caffeine. And if the baby is breast-fed, the supply of caffeine will continue after birth. In this way the baby's caffeine dependence is maintained. But if the baby is formula-fed, the caffeine supply ceases and withdrawal could occur, which could surely contribute to apnea.

The Theory of Caffeine Dependence

Craving for a caffeine-containing beverage often appears specific to particular situations or particular times of the day. For example, a regular coffee drinker may drink a lot of coffee only in the morning and never in the afternoon or evening. Such a person may crave coffee in the mornings but feel no need for it at other times of the day.

This craving may be the result of psychological dependence on caffeine. Psychological dependence is a condition in which the user craves a drug to maintain a sense of well-being and feels discomfort when deprived of it. If this is the only type of dependence involved, one should be able to satisfy the craving by drinking decaffeinated coffee. If the craving includes a physical dependence, drinking decaffeinated coffee would not put off or alleviate the symptoms of caffeine withdrawal. Yet neither type of dependence explains why the lack of caffeine in the afternoon or evening does not lead to withdrawal symptoms.

Experiments with animals and humans have shown that tolerance to a drug can be specific to a particular environment. For example, a person might require less alcohol to become drunk in a strange place than he or she would in the place where alcohol is normally consumed. In this case the person develops a greater tolerance to alcohol when in the familiar environment. The mechanism that is involved is similar to what is called classical conditioning. For example, when a dog is presented with food, it automatically begins to salivate. If a bell is rung every time the dog is fed—thus pairing the sound with the food—after a period of time the animal will salivate just at the ringing of the bell. This new relationship

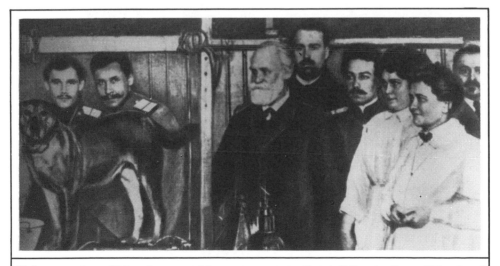

Tolerance to caffeine is caused by a process similar to "classical conditioning," discovered by Russian scientist Ivan Pavlov (center).

between the bell and salivation is the result of classical conditioning. Researchers think that tolerance, too, can be conditioned to be triggered by the events and objects in the environment at the time a drug is taken.

It is generally assumed that tolerance to and physical dependence on a drug go together. If this is true, since tolerance can be explained in part by conditioning, perhaps similar reasoning can be used to explain physical dependence.

Caffeine perks you up. The body, in response to caffeine—perhaps to protect itself from the effects of caffeine—becomes tired and lethargic. This state becomes conditioned to the environment, the events, and even the time of day associated with caffeine use. Thus, when the body is again in the situation in which caffeine is normally used, the conditioned responses of tiredness and lethargy are triggered. The caffeine user experiences these feelings until caffeine is taken.

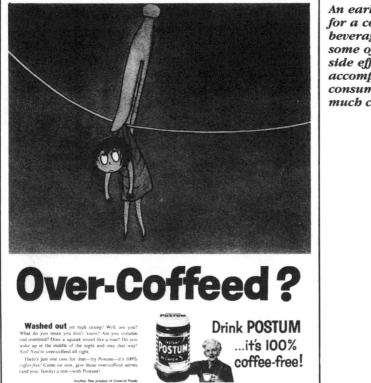

An early advertisement for a coffee-free beverage points out some of the negative side effects that often accompany the consumption of too much caffeine.

If no caffeine is available, the user suffers continued triggering of the unpleasant compensatory responses and experiences a range of withdrawal symptoms.

There is some evidence to support such a theory as it relates to tolerance, but little to show its relationship to drug dependence. However, the above-mentioned account should serve as an illustration of what researchers are thinking about when they attempt to explain drug, and specifically caffeine, dependence.

Caffeine Hangover

As the 1960s had hippies, the late 19th and early 20th century had the Bohemians. Members of this movement, which started in Paris and spread to other European and North American cities, adopted an easygoing, individualistic, and sometimes eccentric life-style which reflected their protest against or indifference to social conventions. According to *Licit and Illicit Drugs,* a book published by Consumers Union,

> *Like today's hippies, the turn-of-the-century bohemians were conspicuously drug-oriented. . . . In addition to alcohol, the bohemians used coffee. They drank vast quantities of this stimulant, were preoccupied with coffee, and suffered coffee as well as alcohol hangovers. Respectable citizens of that era were as horrified by the bohemian coffee cult as today's respectable citizens are horrified by marijuana smoking.*

Although caffeine hangovers are rarely mentioned in medical literature, there is reason to believe that the hangover that follows heavy caffeine use is as real as the hangover that follows heavy alcohol use. Just as the alcohol hangover can to some extent be relieved by more use of alcohol, the physical and emotional depression that sometimes follows a bout of excessive caffeine use can be relieved by use of more caffeine. Rapid intake of 3 or 4 cups of strong coffee provides a severe jolt to the nervous system that causes a high level of arousal and relief from fatigue. Then, some hours later, a headache, mental and physical depression, and feelings of exhaustion result.

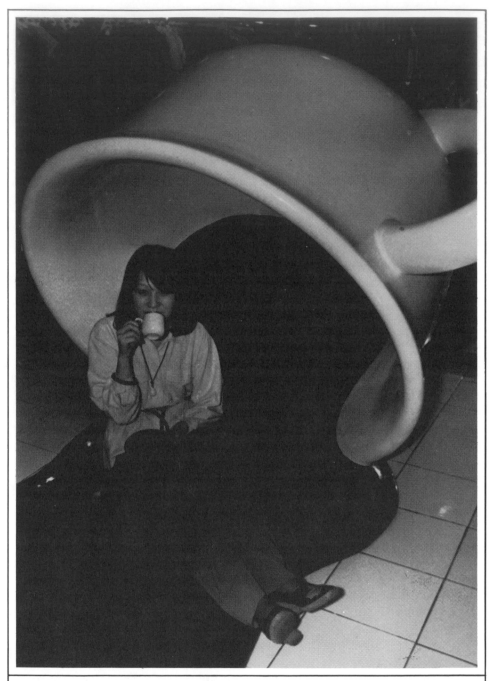

This oversized display in a Tokyo boutique emphasizes the prevalence of coffee in the daily routines of modern society. Although it is difficult to determine what the effects of chronic caffeine use are, sleeplessness and hangover are known to occur frequently.

CHAPTER 10

EFFECTS OF CHRONIC USE OF CAFFEINE

*F*or well over a hundred years there has been medical and popular concern about the effects of the regular use of large amounts of caffeine-containing beverages on mental and physical health. In the late 18th century, William Corbett, author of *The Vice of Tea-Drinking*, wrote that tea drinking is "a destroyer of health, an enfeebler of the frame, an engenderer of effeminacy and laziness, a debaucher of youth, and a maker of misery for old age."

In recent years interest has focused on caffeine's contribution to disease and death from heart conditions and cancer, and on caffeine's role in birth complications and defects. But in fact, there is currently no scientific evidence that suggests that regular use of moderate amounts of caffeine (up to 3 or 4 average cups of coffee per day, or up to about 300 mg of caffeine per day) is harmful to healthy adults. Of course, what constitutes a healthy dose varies according to body weight and many other factors. However, there are three instances that may possibly lead to complications: (1) when caffeine is used by a pregnant woman; (2) when caffeine is regularly consumed in the evening and causes chronic sleeplessness; and (3) when, within a short period of time, a large dose is taken and produces a caffeine hangover that makes the user ill each day.

A Note on Epidemiology

Epidemiology is the branch of medical science concerned with the causes and distribution of disease in populations. It deals with questions such as whether the chances of getting lung cancer increase with the number of cigarettes smoked, and whether the chances of getting typhoid are related to drinking contaminated water from a particular source. Epidemiologists look at a large group of people and attempt to determine how those with a disease differ from those free of the disease. In doing so they hope to be able to pinpoint the factors that could cause the disease.

Epidemiological studies do not by themselves provide scientific proof that a factor contributed to a disease. For example, just because heavy smokers exhibit a high incidence of lung cancer, one cannot immediately conclude that the heavy smoking *caused* the cancer. It might be because heavy smokers tend to live in cities rather than rural areas and it is the urban air pollution that causes lung cancer.

Obviously it is extremely important that epidemiologists consider all the variables and make allowances for them in experiments. In the smoking and lung cancer example, comparing heavy smokers living in cities only with light smokers living in cities would eliminate the variable of residence. But even when it seems that all factors have been considered,

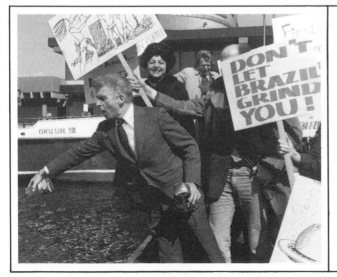

A group of demonstrators dump coffee into New York harbor to protest the sharp rise in Brazilian coffee export taxes, which ballooned 500% in the late 1970s.

there is always the possibility that some unknown variable is the real cause of the disease.

Scientific certainty comes from experiments in which researchers reliably demonstrate a cause-and-effect relationship. Such experiments cannot be done in the case of human disease, because it would be regarded as wholly unethical for scientists to deliberately cause disease in human subjects. Most of our knowledge about the causes of disease, particularly diseases related to life style and drug use, must come from epidemiological work.

A major problem with this kind of research is that much of it relies heavily on reports by the very individuals whose habits are being studied. These reports can be vague or unreliable. Almost all epidemiological studies of caffeine use and disease have relied on information provided by subjects about their usual caffeine-beverage use, generally given in terms of cups of coffee and tea per day. But, as mentioned in Chapter 3, there can be a fourfold range in the caffeine content of six-ounce cups of coffee and tea.

The enormous variability in the meaning of responses to questions about caffeine use is enough to make it almost impossible to find precise relationships between caffeine use and the occurrence of disease. Researchers could develop more accurate indicators of caffeine use by examining blood-caffeine levels or by looking at coffee and tea purchases, but this is usually not done. The general inaccuracy of measures of caffeine use makes it surprising that researchers are willing to give what seem to be unchallengable answers to questions about the extent to which caffeine use contributes to disease.

An important additional complication is the way in which high levels of caffeine use often accompany high levels of other activities, such as smoking, that can also cause disease. Unless researchers isolate caffeine use from other potentially hazardous behaviors, it will continue to be difficult to collect concrete information regarding caffeine's disease-causing effects.

Heart Disease

In the United States heart disease is the leading cause of death. The possibility that heavy caffeine use may contribute to heart disease became a major cause of public concern in the early 1970s, following the announcement of a study that claimed to find a link between heavy coffee drinking (more than six cups a day) and an increased risk of heart attack. This study was shown to be flawed, and the results of a more reliable, longer-term study announced shortly afterward showed no association between coffee consumption and heart attacks or other symptoms of heart disease. However, researchers have continued to explore the possibility of a link.

Three important indicators for heart disease are high blood pressure, arrhythmia (irregular heartbeat), and high blood-cholesterol levels, and caffeine has been studied as a cause of all three. Caffeine has been found to increase blood pressure in subjects who have been without the drug for some days, but tolerance quickly develops to this effect (see Chapters 6 and 8); thus it is unlikely that caffeine would contribute to chronic high blood pressure. On the other hand, heavy caffeine use has been linked to arrhythmias (see Chapter 8) in several studies. One experiment reported that

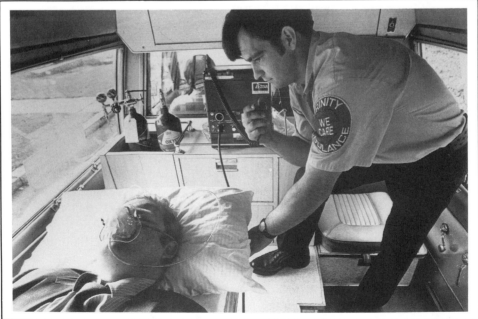

An ambulance technician assists a heart-attack victim en route to the hospital. Although some medical researchers believe that caffeine is a contributor to heart disease, the leading cause of death in the United States, no conclusive evidence of a link has been found.

caffeine produced arrhythmias in subjects who had previous arrhythmic symptoms; another study, or otherwise healthy middle-aged men, found that heavy users of caffeine (more than 8 cups of coffee or tea per day) were more likely than light users (less than 2 cups per day) to exhibit arrhythmia. However, as noted in Chapter 8, a study released in 1989 showed that moderate doses of caffeine (3–4 cups of coffee per day) did not pose a threat even to people with life-threatening arrhythmia. Thus while heavy caffeine consumption has been linked to arrhythmia, light to moderate consumption has little or no effect on the heartbeat.

Some researchers believe that the link between caffeine and heart disease may be found in high cholesterol levels in the blood. Cholesterol, a fatty substance found in cells and fluids, is made by the liver and also obtained from foods derived from animal products—meats, fish, dairy products, and eggs. Cholesterol is a major component of red blood cell membranes and nerve fibers and essential to the proper functioning of the body. However, when too much cholesterol is

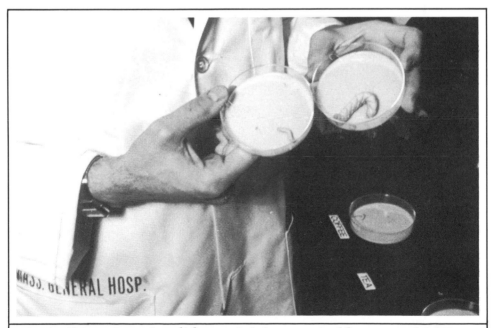

A scientist compares two dishes containing a normal hornworm (right), which was fed its usual diet with a stunted hornworm, which was fed a diet containing a significant amount of caffeine.

present, the excess collects along the walls of the arteries and can cause poor circulation, hardening of the arteries (atherosclerosis), and the formation of blood clots; heart attacks and strokes may result. There are actually two principal forms of cholesterol in the body: HDL and LDL. Researchers now believe that in the healthy body HDL and LDL exist in a delicate balance, with HDL in an amount exceeding that of LDL. The problems resulting from a high cholesterol level in the blood are thought to be caused by an excess of LDL in relation to HDL.

Although caffeine itself does not contain cholesterol—any direct cholesterol consumption via coffee or tea drinking comes from the cream or milk added to the beverage—the drug may be responsible for changes in cholesterol levels in the blood. In 1983 a study of Norwegians found that those drinking more than 9 cups of coffee daily had significantly higher blood cholesterol levels than those drinking less than 1 cup per day. Other studies in the 1970s and early 1980s indicated that cholesterol levels rose in animals who were fed a caffeine-rich diet. More recent research has focused on caffeine and LDL levels, but conflicting results have been reported. In 1989 a study at Stanford University concluded that consuming *decaffeinated* coffee raised LDL levels in middle-aged coffee drinkers who had switched from regular to decaf. The following year a study of coffee drinkers in the Netherlands reported a significant increase in LDL among people who drank boiled coffee; drinkers of filtered coffee—the kind now most commonly consumed in the United States—showed no such effect.

The results of the most recent major study of caffeine and heart disease were reported in the fall of 1990 by the Harvard School of Public Health. Researchers there followed 45,000 men aged 40 to 75 and concluded that coffee drinking, even when heavy, does not make people more likely to develop heart disease or stroke. Research continues in the United States and abroad on this issue, but at present it can be said that no clear and unchallengable evidence supporting a link between caffeine and heart disease exists.

Cancer

The evidence connecting caffeine and cancer is inconclusive. A cancer occurs when cells of the body change in character, begin to divide uncontrollably, and spread to various parts of the body. The change in the cells' character is known as *mutagenesis*, and substances that cause such a change are known as *mutagens*.

As mentioned in Chapter 4, caffeine can interfere with the way in which cells reproduce. Caffeine does this both by reacting directly with and by causing changes in the DNA molecules themselves, and also by interfering with the way DNA reproduces. In this respect caffeine is a mutagen.

Caffeine has been shown to be a mutagen in experimental studies at concentrations that are very much higher than those found in the body after normal caffeine use— typically about 200 times higher. Studies in which caffeine has been shown to be a mutagen have generally been conducted on the cells of bacteria, plants, and insects, and on mammalian cells that have been induced to live and reproduce apart from the whole animal. It is important to note that a substance can change isolated cells without causing cancer in animals and humans.

Lower concentrations of caffeine can enhance the mutagenic effects of other agents, but even these concentrations are at least 6 times the level that would ever occur in a human body after caffeine-beverage use.

Experimental studies on animals have generally *not* found evidence of tumor formation resulting from the long-

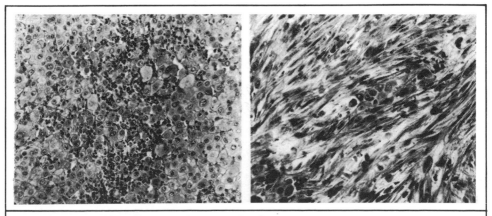

Microphotographs showing the growth of cancer in human tissues. Experiments concerning the correlation between caffeine and cancer have not proved conclusive. In some cases doses of the drug seemed to inhibit tumor production, although at other times caffeine acted as a catalyst.

term administration of high doses of caffeine. When caffeine has been given together with a known carcinogen, the results have been mixed. Large doses administered to animals under carefully controlled conditions have been found to enhance the ability of certain known carcinogens to cause tumors. Similar doses given under different conditions have been found to *inhibit* tumor production. Thus, in combination with known carcinogens, caffeine can be both a carcinogen and an anti-carcinogen.

In analyzing animal studies, one must recognize the possibility that many of the results found in these studies may be irrelevant to studies of diseases in humans because of differences between the metabolism of caffeine in humans and in other species. In humans, the major intermediate metabolite of caffeine, paraxanthine, and the major excretion product, 1-methylxanthine, are both very similar in molecular structure to components of the DNA molecule. Accordingly, both of them may be more likely to interfere with cell reproduction than caffeine itself, although this has not been established. In rats the most important metabolite is a chemical known as 1,3,7-trimethyldihydrouric acid, also found in humans in small quantities. This chemical is *less* similar than the human caffeine metabolites to components of the genetic code. Thus, caffeine ingestion could be carcinogenic in humans and not in rats.

Epidemiological studies conducted in the 1960s and 1970s suggested links between caffeine-beverage use and the development of cancer at the following sites: bladder, kidney, pancreas, colon, prostate gland, breast, and ovary. Later and more carefully conducted studies focused on cancers of the bladder and pancreas, and on cancerous and non-cancerous (benign) tumors of the breast.

Regarding bladder cancer, recent work tends to suggest a link between caffeine-beverage use and deaths from cancer in men, but the evidence for a relationship in women is inconsistent. Positive associations, where found, have been weak but significant. It is reasonable to conclude that heavy coffee use (an average of more than 7 cups per day) can contribute to bladder cancer in men but not necessarily in women. However, overall rates of bladder cancer in women are considerably lower than those in men, making it more difficult to detect a positive relationship.

Recent work concerning pancreatic cancer has produced inconsistent results. Studies have both confirmed and contradicted an earlier finding that linked heavy coffee use and the development of cancer at this site. A British study found an association between heavy use of tea and pancreatic cancer.

However, an epidemiological study can only identify relationships between variables. It cannot determine which of the linked variables is the one most likely to be the causative agent. Therefore, since it is known that damage to the pancreas can lead to increased fluid intake, it is impossible to say if the heavy caffeine use caused the pancreatic cancer or if the pancreatic cancer led to heavy caffeine-beverage use.

A much-publicized 1979 report suggested that benign breast tumors disappeared when caffeine was removed from the diet of women. Subsequent work provides data that do not support this finding, though a link cannot yet be ruled out. Although benign breast tumors can signal the later development of breast cancer, there has been little in the epidemiological studies to suggest a relationship between caffeine-beverage use and breast cancer. Two recent experiments using rats found that the addition of caffeine to their diet enhanced the action of known carcinogens of breast cancer. However, one study found that caffeine tended to prevent the breast cancer in rats caused by the synthetic hormone diethylstilbestrol (DES), used currently as a form of contraception known as "the morning-after pill."

It should be noted that, in studies that found an association between caffeine-beverage use and cancer, the caffeine itself may not be the cause of the cancer. In fact, both tea and coffee contain and are served with other substances that have been identified as mutagens. Therefore, further studies that eliminate the possible role of these other mutagens are needed before caffeine's true role can be known.

"Does caffeine use cause or contribute to cancer in humans?" Presently the answer cannot be a clear "yes" or "no."

Reproductive Problems

Caffeine can affect the unborn child in three distinct ways. First, as an agent that can interfere with the reproduction of cells, caffeine could cause anomalies in sperm or ova, or in the way in which the fertilized ovum divides to form the developing embryo and then the fetus. Second, as a chemical that crosses the placenta, caffeine could directly affect the developing embryo or fetus in many of the ways in which it affects children or adults, or in ways that are especially harmful to an unborn child. And third, caffeine could cause adverse effects in a mother that might have an impact on the development of the unborn child.

Studies in which animals are used as subjects suggest that all three of these things happen. Reviewing the evidence regarding caffeine's effects on reproduction, Beverly Mosher, in her book *The Health Effects of Caffeine*, concluded by saying that,

> *The studies reviewed ... clearly demonstrate that caffeine induces a variety of reproductive effects in several animal systems. Congenital anomalies and reproductive failures, such as reduced fertility, prematurity, low birthweight, and stillbirth have been demonstrated in mice, rats, rabbits, and chickens administered caffeine. Teratological effects [birth*

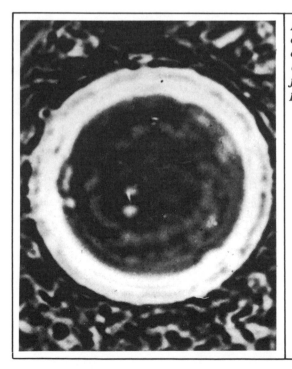

A microphotograph of a human ovum. For some individuals chronic use of caffeine can cause irregularities in the fertilized egg, resulting in possible damage to the fetus.

defects] include cleft palate, digital effects, jaw mal-
formations, missing heart septa, and missing testes.
However, animal tests may not accurately pre-
dict reproductive risk incurred by humans who con-
sume caffeine. No firm guidelines exist for
extrapolating from animal reproductive studies to
humans. Hence, human reproductive risk cannot
be reliably estimated from these animal data. De-
spite these limitations, attempts to define a no-ad-
verse-effect level have been made. The level is
considerably higher than all but the most extreme
human consumption levels. However, certain in-
dividuals with a greater than average sensitivity to
caffeine might also fall into a high-risk category.

When it was written in 1981, this reviewer's conclusion
fairly represented the then current knowledge. In addition
to these findings, caffeine administered to animals during pregnancy had also been found to affect adversely the postnatal
behavior of the offspring. The main effect found in some
studies was an increase in exploratory activity of offspring
or in the general variability of their behavior, neither of which
is necessarily an adverse effect.

Because of the growing number of indications that caffeine could cause reproductive problems, the U.S. Food and
Drug Administration (FDA) began studying caffeine's effects
in the 1970s. In 1978 an FDA committee recommended that
caffeine be removed from the list of substances generally
regarded as safe (the GRAS list). In 1980, prompted further
by its own study of birth defects in rats, the FDA deleted
caffeine from the GRAS list on an interim basis. Further tests
were ordered, and pregnant women were advised "to avoid
caffeine-containing food and drugs, or to use them sparingly."
Canada's federal health department had issued a similar warning in 1979.

The first part of the FDA's own study involved the daily
administration of large single doses of caffeine directly into
the stomachs of pregnant rats. At doses above 25 mg/kg, birth
defects—mainly toe or paw defects—were found in their
offspring.

The second part of the FDA's study involved adding caffeine to the drinking water of pregnant rats. This experiment,
reported in 1983, found no major defects even at the highest

daily dose of 204.5 mg/kg, although reduced birth weight and other problems were reported at doses of 86.6 mg/kg and higher. They reported no effects at or below 51 mg/kg.

Because caffeine administered in rats' drinking water is more like human caffeine-beverage consumption than administration directly into the stomach by a tube, and because the former route was found to be less hazardous, the FDA continues to assess its position on caffeine. Moderation may remain part of the FDA's advice, said a spokesman, because "caffeine is a drug no matter how you slice it. ... [Pregnant] women ought to limit their intake, but don't have to think they can't drink any caffeine or colas."

But how does one relate a daily dose of 50 mg/kg in rats' drinking water to a safe level for a pregnant woman? Some scientists have suggested that a 100:1 safety factor should be used in extrapolating the results of animal studies of birth defects. This would mean that the safe daily dose of caffeine for a pregnant woman would be that found in about half of an average cup of coffee. A second group of researchers has suggested that the correct conversion factor between rats and humans is 4:1, meaning that the safe daily dose for pregnant women would be the equivalent of about 7 strong cups of coffee. A third group of researchers believes that a 1:1 conversion is appropriate, meaning that the safety limit would be about 28 strong cups of coffee. If this were true pregnant women could essentially drink as much coffee as they pleased without adverse effect on their unborn children.

Studies of the relation between caffeine use and human birth defects and problems have generally not produced conclusive results. Part of the problem is that pregnant women tend to reduce their caffeine use during pregnancy (see Chapter 5), making it difficult to find enough heavy caffeine users to make up a significant sample.

One study attempted to overcome this problem by interviewing 12,205 women about their coffee and tea consumption during the first three months of their pregnancies and relating this to the incidence of birth difficulties and defects. Only 595 of these women (4.9% of the total) reported drinking 4 or more cups of coffee per day. The babies of these heavy coffee users tended to be premature and lighter than average and were more likely to be born breech first rather than head first. However, this study failed to control for cigarette use, which was common among these heavy coffee drinkers.

Two other recent studies compared the caffeine use by women who had given birth to malformed infants with that of women who had had normal babies. In a U.S. study that compared 2,030 such pairs, malformed infants were slightly more likely to have had mothers who had used some caffeine during pregnancy. However, the differences were not statistically significant and the estimated risk was not higher with high levels of caffeine use. A similar Finnish study involving 755 pairs showed no evidence of increased risk with caffeine use, even though average levels of consumption were very much higher than those in the United States.

One can only conclude that at the moment there is no direct evidence that high levels of caffeine ingested during pregnancy give rise to birth difficulties and defects. Evidence

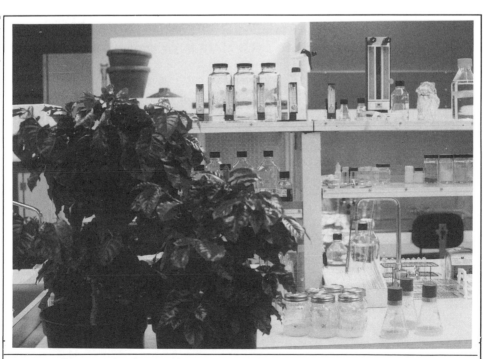

A laboratory at the Escagenetics Corporation, a West Coast biotechnology company. Scientists at the company announced in 1990 that they are developing a coffee plant that produces low-caffeine beans.

from animal studies, however, supports the conclusion that during pregnancy it is wise for women to be cautious about consuming caffeine in any form.

Behavioral Disorders: Caffeinism

Chronic excessive caffeine use has long been associated with abnormal behavior. There was renewed interest in this possibility in the 1970s and early 1980s with the appearance of a number of reports that psychiatric patients with high levels of anxiety often drank a lot of coffee and could decrease their anxiety by reducing their caffeine intake.

In one study, for example, 22% of hospitalized psychiatric patients, whose scores on tests for anxiety and depression were significantly higher than normal, were found to be excessive users of caffeine (750 mg or more per day). In another study, 14 male psychiatric patients were, unknown to them or their nurses, given decaffeinated rather than regular coffee for 3 weeks. Tests showed a reduction in anxiety, irritability, suspiciousness, and hostility. When regular coffee was introduced, previous levels of these psychological problems returned.

The syndrome, or group of symptoms, associated with excessive caffeine use is known as *caffeinism*. John Greden, psychiatrist, has written:

> *The most common anxiety manifestations of caffeinism are frequent urination (caffeine diuresis), jitteriness, tremulousness, agitation, irritability, muscle twitchings, lightheadedness, rapid breathing (tachypnea), rapid heart beat (tachycardia), cardiac palpitations (or skipped beats), upset stomach, loose stools and epigastric distress (heartburn and similar pains). Seldom do all occur together. ... clinicians may find it impossible to differentiate the condition from anxiety neurosis or situational anxiety.*

Many of these symptoms of caffeinism are consequences of the acute use of caffeine described in Chapters 8 and 9. The caffeinism syndrome appears to be a chronic problem because the patients are chronically anxious, i.e., they are anxious every day. But they may be anxious every day only because they use large amounts of caffeine every day.

Excessive caffeine use and stress have similar effects on the body. When they occur simultaneously their effects may be additive. Animal studies have shown that caffeine worsens both gastric ulceration and kidney disease when these conditions are caused by stress. Animals living in crowded circumstances show increased aggression when given caffeine. However, caffeine has also been found to *reduce* aggressiveness in rats that have been in isolation.

In humans, the combination of caffeine and competitive stress has been reported to cause delirium. Caffeine and emotional stress have been reported as causing higher-than-usual levels of adrenaline in the body. Interestingly, increased caffeine-beverage use can be a response to stress. One study found that female (but not male) college students used considerably more caffeine than normal during the week of their final examinations. The combination could have caused serious interference with sleep and excessive arousal, both of which could have interfered with good performance.

Caffeine has also been found to interfere with relaxation training, which is used to reduce a patient's reaction to stress. Caffeine-using subjects learned to relax just as easily as caffeine-free subjects. But, unlike the caffeine-free subjects, the caffeine users were unable to maintain a state of relaxation while viewing a stressful film.

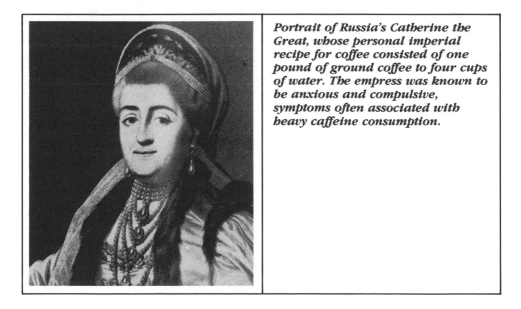

Portrait of Russia's Catherine the Great, whose personal imperial recipe for coffee consisted of one pound of ground coffee to four cups of water. The empress was known to be anxious and compulsive, symptoms often associated with heavy caffeine consumption.

One of the problems with treating caffeinism is that caffeine withdrawal itself can be stressful (see Chapter 9). A patient who is chronically anxious as a result of using caffeine may become more anxious when caffeine is withdrawn, and the anxiety may be made worse by a withdrawal headache.

Finally, the small amount of evidence specifically related to children suggests that they respond to caffeine just as adults do. If children regularly use large doses of caffeine they can become chronically irritable, restless, and anxious. These symptoms can also occur in asthmatic children who are being treated with large doses of theophylline.

Some children appear to be calmed rather than aroused by stimulant drugs. These children have been described as suffering from hyperactivity (variously known as hyperkinesis, excessive motor restlessness, and attention deficit disorder), learning disabilities, or even minimal brain dysfunction. One explanation of this paradox is that such children are hyperactive because their nervous systems are naturally under-aroused. In other words, they move around a lot, speak out, and are generally disruptive in class because

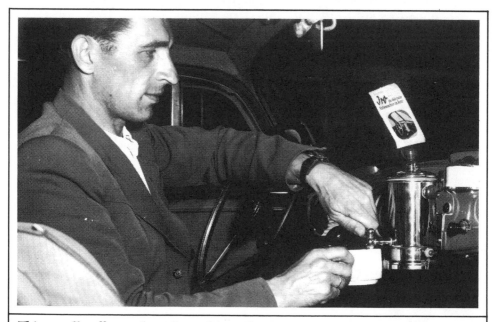

This small coffee maker plugged into the dashboard of a car—suggesting that coffee was just as popular in the 1950s as it is today.

they need to keep themselves from becoming lethargic or falling asleep. According to this theory, stimulant drugs provide this arousal of the nervous system, making the hyperactivity unnecessary.

This theory is similar to the explanation for the different effects of caffeine on impulsive and nonimpulsive people (see Chapter 7). However, neither theory is based on actual measurements of the arousal levels of the nervous systems of different adults and children.

Amphetamines, the stimulant drugs usually given to such children, are reported to help most hyperactive youngsters, although unwanted side effects have been reported. Some clinicians have used caffeine as an alternative. Experimental studies of caffeine's effectiveness have produced contradictory results. One study found that hyperactive children who used methylphenidate, a type of amphetamine, exhibited significantly improved behavior, whereas caffeine (300 mg or 500 mg per day) produced no effect. Another study found that a lower dose of caffeine (about 150 mg) together with a low dose of methylphenidate (10 mg) was more effective than the low dose of methylphenidate alone, while a higher dose of caffeine (about 300 mg) with the methylphenidate dose was not effective in improving behavior.

Thus, one can see that though caffeine can calm some children, it makes most children more restless, irritable, and anxious. Clearly, more research is necessary before caffeine can be used to provide consistent and predictable responses in children.

Hazardous Levels of Chronic Caffeine Use

According to the studies mentioned in this chapter, regular use of more than about 650 mg of caffeine (8 or more cups of coffee per day, or 14 cans of Coke) may be associated with higher incidences of ventricular premature heartbeats (irregular heartbeats), high levels of cholesterol, bladder cancer (in men), and behavioral disorders. And while some researchers consider this dose as the maximum which can be used safely by a pregnant woman, many others have argued for a lower level and a few have argued for a higher level.

Given the most current evidence, it is reasonable to conclude that, in general, healthy adults may consume up to 600 mg of caffeine per day without doing themselves harm.

As mentioned earlier, caffeine use during pregnancy, use that leads to chronic sleeplessness, and use of high doses that lead to hangover may be exceptions. Also, it follows that since physical dependence on caffeine can occur at doses of approximately 400 mg per day, a person may be dependent on caffeine without necessarily being at risk of being affected by the various diseases that have been associated with caffeine use.

Approximately 3% of North Americans aged 15 years and over, or at least 6 million people, use 650 mg or more caffeine per day and thus are putting themselves at risk. Another 30 million or so have some kind of dependence on caffeine, a condition which may or may not be hazardous.

The risk from excessive caffeine use should not be exaggerated. Although it is possible to say with some confidence that excessive caffeine use is harmful, the harm is probably slight compared with that resulting from excessive use of alcohol or almost any use of tobacco.

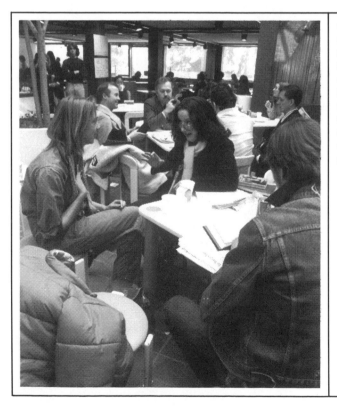

College women enjoy a cup of coffee between classes. According to one study, female college students used much higher amounts of caffeine during the stressful week of examinations than did their male counterparts.

Conclusion

Because caffeine is a relatively weak drug, but one that affects many parts of the body, sorting out the many consequences of using it have presented researchers with special difficulties. When humans are being studied, these difficulties are compounded by the pervasiveness of caffeine in our society. Because almost everyone uses caffeine and has experienced its effects, there are few unbiased or naive subjects.

Caffeine is used for its beneficial short-term effects—usually to maintain or increase alertness and to enhance physical endurance. About one in four North American adults may be dependent on caffeine and use it at least in part to ward off withdrawal symptoms. And about 1 in 30 adults may regularly use enough caffeine to cause physical harm. Of special concern is the possibility that caffeine used during pregnancy may cause or contribute to birth defects and difficulties. This possibility led the U.S. Food and Drug Administration to delete caffeine in 1980 from the list of drugs generally regarded as safe. Caffeine is a drug, and though present data regarding its safety may be inconclusive, it is wise to use it cautiously and in moderation.

Appendix I

POPULATION ESTIMATES OF LIFETIME AND CURRENT NONMEDICAL DRUG USE, 1988

	12-17 years (pop. 20,250,000)		18-25 years (pop. 29,688,000)	
	% Ever Used	% Current User	% Ever Used	% Current User
Marijuana & Hashish	17 3,516,000	6 1,296,000	56 16,741,000	16 4,594,000
Hallucinogens	3 704,000	1 168,000	14 4,093,000	2 569,000
Inhalants	9 1,774,000	2 410,000	12 3,707,000	2 514,000
Cocaine	3 683,000	1 225,000	20 5,858,000	5 1,323,000
Crack	1 188,000	+ +	3 1,000,000	1 249,000
Heroin	1 118,000	+ +	+ +	+ +
Stimulants*	4 852,000	1 245,000	1 3,366,000	2 718,000
Sedatives	2 475,000	1 1 23,000	6 1,633,000	1 265,000
Tranquilizers	2 413,000	+ +	8 2,319,000	1 307,000
Analgesics	4 840,000	1 182,000	9 2,798,000	1 440,000
Alcohol	50 10,161,000	25 5,097,000	90 26,807,000	65 19,392,000
Cigarettes	42 8,564,000	12 2,389,000	75 22,251,000	35 10,447,000
Smokeless Tobacco	15 3,021,000	4 722,000	24 6,971,000	6 1,855,000

* Amphetamines and related substances
+ Amounts of less than .5% are not listed
  Terms: Ever Used: used at least once in a person's lifetime.
       Current User: used at least once in the 30 days prior to the survey.

Source: National Institute on Drug Abuse, August 1989

POPULATION ESTIMATES OF LIFETIME AND CURRENT NONMEDICAL DRUG USE, 1988

26+ years (pop. 148,409,000)				TOTAL (pop. 198,347,000)			
%	Ever Used	%	Current User	%	Ever Used	%	Current User
31	45,491,000	4	5,727,000	33	65,748,000	6	11,616,000
7	9,810,000	+	+	7	4,607,000	+	+
4	5,781,000	+	+	6	1,262,000	1	1,223,000
10	14,631,000	1	1,375,000	11	21,171,000	2	2,923,000
+	+	+	+	1	2,483,000	+	484,000
1	1,686,000	+	+	1	1,907,000	+	+
7	9,850,000	1	791,000	7	4,068,000	1	1,755,000
3	4,867,000	+	+	4	6,975,000	+	+
5	6,750,000	1	822,000	5	9,482,000	1	1,174,000
5	6,619,000	+	+	5	10,257,000	1	1,151,000
89	131,530,000	55	81,356,000	85	168,498,000	53	105,845,000
80	118,191,000	30	44,284,000	75	149,005,000	29	57,121,000
13	19,475,000	3	4,497,000	15	29,467,000	4	7,073,000

Appendix II

DRUGS MENTIONED MOST FREQUENTLY BY HOSPITAL EMERGENCY ROOMS, 1988

	Drug name	Number of mentions by emergency rooms	Percent of total number of mentions
1	Cocaine	62,141	38.80
2	Alcohol-in-combination	46,588	29.09
3	Heroin/Morphine	20,599	12.86
4	Marijuana/Hashish	10,722	6.69
5	PCP/PCP Combinations	8,403	5.25
6	Acetaminophen	6,426	4.01
7	Diazepam	6,082	3.80
8	Aspirin	5,544	3.46
9	Ibuprofen	3,878	2.42
10	Alprazolam	3,846	2.40
11	Methamphetamine/Speed	3,030	1.89
12	Acetaminophen W Codeine	2,457	1.53
13	Amitriptyline	1,960	1.22
14	D.T.C. Sleep Aids	1,820	1.14
15	Methadone	1,715	1.07
16	Triazolam	1,640	1.02
17	Diphenhydramine	1,574	0.98
18	D-Propoxyphene	1,563	0.98
19	Hydantoin	1,442	0.90
20	Lorazepam	1,345	0.84
21	LSD	1,317	0.82
22	Amphetamine	1,316	0.82
23	Phenobarbital	1,223	0.76
24	Oxycodone	1,192	0.74
25	Imipramine	1,064	0.66

Source: Drug Abuse Warning Network (DAWN), Annual Data 1988

Appendix III

DRUGS MENTIONED MOST FREQUENTLY BY MEDICAL EXAMINERS (IN AUTOPSY REPORTS), 1988

	Drug name	Number of mentions in autopsy reports	Percent of total number of drug mentions
1	Cocaine	3,308	48.96
2	Alcohol-in-combination	2,596	38.43
3	Heroin/Morphine	2,480	36.71
4	Codeine	689	10.20
5	Diazepam	464	6.87
6	Methadone	447	6.62
7	Amitriptyline	402	5.95
8	Nortriptyline	328	4.85
9	Lidocaine	306	4.53
10	Acetaminophen	293	4.34
11	D-Propoxyphene	271	4.01
12	Marijuana/Hashish	263	3.89
13	Quinine	224	3.32
14	Unspec Benzodiazepine	222	3.29
15	PCP/PCP Combinations	209	3.09
16	Diphenhydramine	192	2.84
17	Phenobarbital	183	2.71
18	Desipramine	177	2.62
19	Methamphetamine/Speed	161	2.38
20	Doxepin	152	2.25
21	Aspirin	138	2.04
22	Imipramine	137	2.03
23	Hydantoin	98	1.45
24	Amphetamine	87	1.29
25	Chlordiazepoxide	76	1.12

Source: Drug Abuse Warning Network (DAWN), Annual Data 1988

Appendix IV

NATIONAL HIGH SCHOOL SENIOR SURVEY, 1975-1989

	High School Senior Survey Trends in Lifetime Prevalence Percent Who Ever Used				
	Class of 1975	Class of 1976	Class of 1977	Class of 1978	Class of 1979
Marijuana/Hashish	47.3	52.8	56.4	59.2	60.4
Inhalants	NA	10.3	11.1	12.0	12.7
Inhalants Adjusted	NA	NA	NA	NA	18.2
Amyl & Butyl Nitrites	NA	NA	NA	NA	11.1
Hallucinogens	16.3	15.1	13.9	14.3	14.1
Hallucinogens Adjusted	NA	NA	NA	NA	17.7
LSD	11.3	11.0	9.8	9.7	9.5
PCP	NA	NA	NA	NA	12.8
Cocaine	9.0	9.7	10.8	12.9	15.4
Crack	NA	NA	NA	NA	NA
Other cocaine	NA	NA	NA	NA	NA
Heroin	2.2	1.8	1.8	1.6	1.1
Other Opiates*	9.0	9.6	10.3	9.9	10.1
Stimulants*	22.3	22.6	23.0	22.9	24.2
Stimulants Adjusted*	NA	NA	NA	NA	NA
Sedatives*	18.2	17.7	17.4	16.0	14.6
Barbiturates*	16.9	16.2	15.6	13.7	11.8
Methaqualone*	8.1	7.8	8.5	7.9	8.3
Tranquilizers*	17.0	16.8	18.0	17.0	16.3
Alcohol	90.4	91.9	92.5	93.1	93.0
Cigarettes	73.6	75.4	75.7	75.3	74.0

Stimulants adjusted to exclude inappropriate reporting of nonprescription stimulants; stimulants = amphetamines and amphetamine-like substances.
*Only use not under a doctor's orders included.

Source: National Institute on Drug Abuse, National High School Senior Survey: "Monitoring the Future," 1989

NATIONAL HIGH SCHOOL SENIOR SURVEY, 1975-1989

High School Senior Survey
Trends in Lifetime Prevalence
Percent Who Ever Used

Class of 1980	Class of 1981	Class of 1982	Class of 1983	Class of 1984	Class of 1985	Class of 1986	Class of 1987	Class of 1988	Class of 1989
60.3	59.5	58.7	57.0	54.9	54.2	50.9	50.2	47.2	43.7
11.9	12.3	12.8	13.6	14.4	15.4	15.9	17.0	16.7	17.6
17.3	17.2	17.7	18.2	18.0	18.1	20.1	18.6	17.5	18.6
11.1	10.1	9.8	8.4	8.1	7.9	8.6	4.7	3.2	3.3
13.3	13.3	12.5	11.9	10.7	10.3	9.7	10.3	8.9	9.4
15.6	15.3	14.3	13.6	12.3	12.1	11.9	10.6	9.2	9.9
9.3	9.8	9.6	8.9	8.0	7.5	7.2	8.4	7.7	8.3
9.6	7.8	6.0	5.6	5.0	4.9	4.8	3.0	2.9	3.9
15.7	16.5	16.0	16.2	16.1	17.3	16.9	15.2	12.1	10.3
NA	NA	NA	NA	NA	NA	NA	5.4	4.8	4.7
NA	NA	NA	NA	NA	NA	NA	14.0	12.1	8.5
1.1	1.1	1.2	1.2	1.3	1.2	1.1	1.2	1.1	1.3
9.8	10.1	9.6	9.4	9.7	10.2	9.0	9.2	8.6	8.3
26.4	32.2	35.6	35.4	NA	NA	NA	NA	NA	NA
NA	NA	27.9	26.9	27.9	26.2	23.4	21.6	19.8	19.1
14.9	16.0	15.2	14.4	13.3	11.8	10.4	8.7	7.8	7.4
11.0	11.3	10.3	9.9	9.9	9.2	8.4	7.4	6.7	6.5
9.5	10.6	10.7	10.1	8.3	6.7	5.2	4.0	3.3	2.7
15.2	14.7	14.0	13.3	12.4	11.9	10.9	10.9	9.4	7.6
93.2	92.6	92.8	92.6	92.6	92.2	91.3	92.2	92.0	90.7
71.0	71.0	70.1	70.6	69.7	68.8	67.6	67.2	66.4	65.7

Appendix V

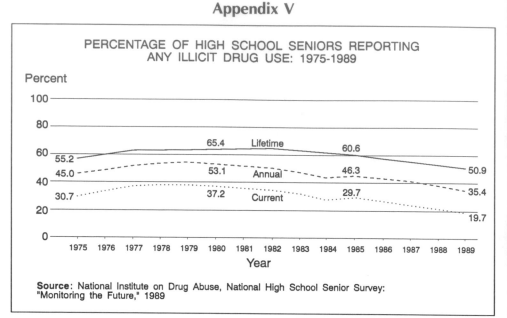

PERCENTAGE OF HIGH SCHOOL SENIORS REPORTING
ANY ILLICIT DRUG USE: 1975-1989

Source: National Institute on Drug Abuse, National High School Senior Survey: "Monitoring the Future," 1989

Appendix VI

DRUG ABUSE AND AIDS

An estimated 25 percent of all cases of acquired immunodeficiency syndrome, or AIDS, are intravenous (IV) drug abusers. This group is the second largest at risk for AIDS, exceeded only by homosexual, and bisexual men. And the numbers may be growing. Data for the first half of 1988 show that IV drug abusers made up about 31 percent of the total reported cases.

". . . the number of IV drug users with AIDS is doubling every 14-16 months."

According to the National Institute on Drug Abuse (NIDA). There are 1.1 to 1.3 million IV drug users in the United States, and, so far, about 17,500 have developed AIDS. Thousands more are infected with the virus that causes this fatal illness, which kills by destroying the body's ability to fight disease.

Currently, the number of IV drug users with AIDS is doubling every 14-16 months. Although the numbers of IV drug users who carry the AIDS virus varies from region to region, in some places the majority may already be infected. In New York City, for example, 60 percent of IV drug users entering treatment programs have the AIDS virus.

Among IV drug abusers, the AIDS virus is spread primarily by needle sharing. As long as IV drug abusers are drug dependent, they are likely to engage in needle sharing. Thus, the key to eliminating needle sharing—and the associated spread of AIDS—is drug abuse treatment to curb drug dependence. NIDA is working to find ways to get more IV users into treatment and to develop new methods to fight drug addiction. Most non-drug users characteristically associate heroin with IV drug use. However, thousands of others inject cocaine or amphetamines. Recent evidence suggests that IV cocaine use is increasing and that the AIDS virus is spreading in those users. One reason for this may be because cocaine's effects last only a short time. When the drug, which is a stimulant, wears off, users may inject again and again, sharing a needle many times in a few hours. In contrast, heroin users inject once and fall asleep.

". . . IV cocaine use is increasing and the AIDS virus is spreading in those users."

The apparent increase in IV cocaine is especially worrisome, drug abuse experts say, because there are no standard therapies for treating cocaine addiction. Until scientists find effective treatments for this problem, the ability to control the spread of AIDS will be hampered.

TRANSMISSION

Needle Sharing -- Among IV drug users, transmission of AIDS virus most often occurs by sharing needles, syringes, or other "works." Small amounts of contaminated blood left in the equipment can carry the virus from user to user. IV drug abusers who frequent "shooting galleries" — where paraphernalia is passed among several people -- are at especially high risk for AIDS. But, needle sharing of any sort (at parties, for example) can transmit the virus, and NIDA experts note that almost all IV drug users share needles at one time or another.
Because not every IV drug abuser will enter treatment and because some must wait to be treated, IV users in many cities are being taught to flush their "works" with bleach before they inject. Used correctly, bleach can destroy virus left in the equipment.

Sexual Transmission -- IV drug abusers also get AIDS through unprotected sex with someone who is infected. In addition, the AIDS virus can be sexually transmitted from infected IV drug abusers to individuals who do not use drugs. Data from the Centers for Disease Control show that IV drug use is associated with the increased spread of AIDS in the heterosexual population. For example, of all women reported to have AIDS, 49 percent were IV drug users, while another 30 percent -- non-IV drug users themselves -- were sexual partners of IV drug users. Infected women who become pregnant can pass the AIDS virus to their babies. About 70 percent of all children born with AIDS have had a mother or father who shot drugs.

Non-IV Drug Use and AIDS -- Sexual activity has also been reported as the means of AIDS transmission among those who use non-IV drugs (like crack or marijuana). Many people, especially women, addicted to crack (or other substances) go broke supporting their habit and turn to trading sex for drugs. Another link between substance abuse and AIDS is when individuals using alcohol and drugs relax their restraints and caution regarding sexual behavior. People who normally practice "safe" sex may neglect to do so while "under the influence."

Source: U.S. Public Health Service, AIDS Program Office, 1989

Appendix VII

U.S. Drug Schedules*

	Drugs Included	Dispensing Regulations
Schedule I high potential for abuse; no currently accepted medical use in treatment in U.S.; safety not proven for medical use	heroin methaqualone LSD mescaline peyote phencyclidine analogs psilocybin marijuana hashish	research use only
Schedule II high potential for abuse; currently accepted U.S. medical use; abuse may lead to severe psychological or physical dependence	opium morphine methadone barbiturates cocaine amphetamines phencyclidine codeine	written Rx; no refills
Schedule III less potential for abuse than drugs in Schedules I and II; currently accepted U.S. medical use; may lead to moderate or low physical dependence or high psychological dependence	glutethimide selected morphine, opium, and codeine compounds selected depressant sedative compounds selected stimulants for weight control	written or oral Rx; refills allowed
Schedule IV low potential for abuse relative to drugs in Schedule III; currently accepted U.S. medical use; abuse may lead to limited physical dependence or psychological dependence relative to drugs in Schedule III	selected barbiturate and other depressant compounds selected stimulants for weight control	written or oral Rx; refills allowed
Schedule V low potential for abuse relative to drugs in Schedule IV; currently accepted U.S. medical use; abuse may lead to limited physical dependence or psychological dependence relative to drugs in Schedule IV	selected narcotic compounds	OTC/ M.D.'s order

*Established by the U.S. Controlled Substances Act of 1970
Source: U.S. Drug Enforcement Administration

Appendix VIII

Agencies for the Prevention and Treatment of Drug Abuse

UNITED STATES

Alabama
Department of Mental Health
Division of Substance Abuse
200 Interstate Park Drive
P.O. Box 3710
Montgomery, AL 36109
(205) 270-9650

Alaska
Department of Health and
Social Services
Division of Alcoholism and
Drug Abuse
P.O. Box H
Juneau, AK 99811-0607
(907) 586-6201

Arizona
Department of Health
Services
Division of Behavioral Health
Services
Bureau of Community
Services
The Office of Substance
Abuse
2632 East Thomas
Phoenix, AZ 85016
(602) 255-1030

Arkansas
Department of Human
Services
Division of Alcohol and Drug
Abuse
400 Donagy Plaza North
P.O. Box 1437
Slot 2400
Little Rock, AR 72203-1437
(501) 682-6656

California
Health and Welfare Agencies
Department of Alcohol and
Drug Programs
1700 K Street
Sacramento, CA 95814-4037
(916) 445-1943

Colorado
Department of Health
Alcohol and Drug Abuse
Division
4210 East 11th Avenue
Denver, CO 80220
(303) 331-8201

Connecticut
Alcohol and Drug Abuse
Commission
999 Asylum Avenue
3rd Floor
Hartford, CT 06105
(203) 566-4145

Delaware
Division of Mental Health
Bureau of Alcoholism and
Drug Abuse
1901 North Dupont Highway
Newcastle, DE 19720
(302) 421-6101

District of Columbia
Department of Human
Services
Office of Health Planning and
Development
1660 L Street NW
Room 715
Washington, DC 20036
(202) 724-5641

Florida
Department of Health and
Rehabilitative Services
Alcohol, Drug Abuse, and
Mental Health Office
1317 Winewood Boulevard
Building 6, Room 183
Tallahassee, FL 32399-0700
(904) 488-8304

Georgia
Department of Human
Resources
Division of Mental Health,
Mental Retardation, and
Substance Abuse
Alcohol and Drug Section
878 Peachtree Street
Suite 319
Atlanta, GA 30309-3917
(404) 894-4785

Hawaii
Department of Health
Mental Health Division
Alcohol and Drug Abuse
Branch
1270 Queen Emma Street
Room 706
Honolulu, HI 96813
(808) 548-4280

Idaho
Department of Health and
Welfare
Bureau of Preventive
Medicine
Substance Abuse Section
450 West State
Boise, ID 83720
(208) 334-5934

Illinois
Department of Alcoholism
and Substance Abuse
Illinois Center
100 West Randolph Street
Suite 5-600
Chicago, IL 60601
(312) 814-3840

Indiana
Department of Mental Health
Division of Addiction Services
117 East Washington Street
Indianapolis, IN 46204-3647
(317) 232-7816

Iowa
Department of Public Health
Division of Substance Abuse
Lucas State Office Building
321 East 12th Street
Des Moines, IA 50319
(515) 281-3641

Kansas
Department of Social
  Rehabilitation
Alcohol and Drug Abuse
  Services
300 SW Oakley
2nd Floor
Biddle Building
Topeka, KS 66606
(913) 296-3925

Kentucky
Cabinet for Human Resources
Department of Health
  Services
Substance Abuse Branch
275 East Main Street
Frankfort, KY 40621
(502) 564-2880

Louisiana
Department of Health and
  Hospitals
Office of Human Services
Division of Alcohol and Drug
  Abuse
P.O. Box 3868
Baton Rouge, LA 70821-3868
1201 Capital Access Road
Baton Rouge, LA 70802
(504) 342-9354

Maine
Department of Human
  Services
Office of Alcoholism and
  Drug Abuse Prevention
Bureau of Rehabilitation
5 Anthony Avenue
State House, Station 11
Augusta, ME 04433
(207) 289-2781

Maryland
Alcohol and Drug Abuse
  Administration
201 West Preston Street

4th Floor
Baltimore, MD 21201
(301) 225-6910

Massachusetts
Department of Public Health
Division of Substance Abuse
150 Tremont Street
Boston, MA 02111
(617) 727-1960

Michigan
Department of Public Health
Office of Substance Abuse
  Services
2150 Apollo Drive
P.O. Box 30206
Lansing, MI 48909
(517) 335-8810

Minnesota
Department of Human
  Services
Chemical Dependency
  Division
444 Lafayette Road
St. Paul, MN 55155
(612) 296-4614

Mississippi
Department of Mental Health
Division of Alcohol and Drug
  Abuse
1101 Robert E. Lee Building
239 North Lamar Street
Jackson, MS 39201
(601) 359-1288

Missouri
Department of Mental
  Health
Division of Alcoholism and
  Drug Abuse
1706 East Elm Street
P.O. Box 687
Jefferson City, MO 65102
(314) 751-4942

Montana
Department of Institutions
Alcohol and Drug Abuse
  Division
1539 11th Avenue
Helena, MT 59620
(406) 444-2827

Nebraska
Department of Public
  Institutions
Division of Alcoholism and
  Drug Abuse
801 West Van Dorn Street
P.O. Box 94728
Lincoln, NB 68509-4728
(402) 471-2851, Ext. 5583

Nevada
Department of Human
  Resources
Bureau of Alcohol and Drug
  Abuse
505 East King Street
Room 500
Carson City, NV 89710
(702) 687-4790

New Hampshire
Department of Health and
  Human Services
Office of Alcohol and Drug
  Abuse Prevention
State Office
Park South
105 Pleasant Street
Concord, NH 03301
(603) 271-6100

New Jersey
Department of Health
Division of Alcoholism and
  Drug Abuse
129 East Hanover Street CN
  362
Trenton, NJ 08625
(609) 292-8949

New Mexico
Health and Environment
  Department
Behavioral Health Services
  Division/
Substance Abuse
Harold Runnels Building
1190 Saint Francis Drive
Santa Fe, NM 87503
(505) 827-2601

New York
Division of Alcoholism and
  Alcohol Abuse
194 Washington Avenue

Albany, NY 12210
(518) 474-5417

Division of Substance Abuse
    Services
Executive Park South
Box 8200
Albany, NY 12203
(518) 457-7629

North Carolina
Department of Human
    Resources
Division of Mental Health,
    Developmental Disabilities,
    and Substance Abuse
    Services
Alcohol and Drug Abuse
    Services
325 North Salisbury Street
Albemarle Building
Raleigh, NC 27603
(919) 733-4670

North Dakota
Department of Human
    Services
Division of Alcohol and Drug
    Abuse
1839 East Capital Avenue
Bismarck, ND 58501-2152
(701) 224-2769

Ohio
Division of Alcohol and Drug
    Addiction Services
246 North High Street
Columbus, OH 43266-0170
(614) 466-3445

Oklahoma
Department of Mental Health
    and Substance Abuse
    Services
Alcohol and Drug Abuse
    Services
1200 North East 13th Street
P.O. Box 53277
Oklahoma City, OK 73152-
    3277
(405) 271-8653

Oregon
Department of Human
    Resources

Office of Alcohol and Drug
    Abuse Programs
1178 Chemeketa NE
#102
Salem, OR 97310
(503) 378-2163

Pennsylvania
Department of Health
Office of Drug and Alcohol
    Programs
Health and Welfare Building
Room 809
P.O. Box 90
Harrisburg, PA 17108
(717) 787-9857

Rhode Island
Department of Mental Health,
    Mental Retardation and
    Hospitals
Division of Substance Abuse
Substance Abuse
    Administration Building
P.O. Box 20363
Cranston, RI 02920
(401) 464-2091

South Carolina
Commission on Alcohol and
    Drug Abuse
3700 Forest Drive
Suite 300
Columbia, SC 29204
(803) 734-9520

South Dakota
Department of Human Services
700 Governor's Drive
Pier South D
Pierre, SD 57501-2291
(605) 773-4806

Tennessee
Department of Mental Health
    and Mental Retardation
Alcohol and Drug Abuse
    Services
706 Church Street
Nashville, TN 37243-0675
(615) 741-1921

Texas
Commission on Alcohol and
    Drug Abuse

720 Bracos Street
Suite 403
Austin, TX 78701
(512) 463-5510

Utah
Department of Social Services
Division of Substance Abuse
120 North 200 West
4th Floor
Salt Lake City, UT 84103
(801) 538-3939

Vermont
Agency of Human Services
Department of Social and
    Rehabilitation Services
Office of Alcohol and Drug
    Abuse Programs
103 South Main Street
Waterbury, VT 05676
(802) 241-2170

Virginia
Department of Mental Health
    and Mental Retardation
Division of Substance Abuse
109 Governor Street
8th Floor
P.O. Box 1797
Richmond, VA 23214
(804) 786-5313

Washington
Department of Social and
    Health Service
Division of Alcohol and
    Substance Abuse
12th and Franklin
Mail Stop OB 21W
Olympia, WA 98504
(206) 753-5866

West Virginia
Department of Health and
    Human Resources
Office of Behavioral Health
    Services
Division on Alcoholism and
    Drug Abuse
Capital Complex
1900 Kanawha Boulevard East
Building 3, Room 402
Charleston, WV 25305
(304) 348-2276

Wisconsin
Department of Health and
  Social Services
Division of Community
  Services
Bureau of Community
  Programs
Office of Alcohol and Drug
  Abuse
1 West Wilson Street
P.O. Box 7851
Madison, WI 53707-7851
(608) 266-2717

Wyoming
Alcohol And Drug Abuse
  Programs
451 Hathaway Building
Cheyenne, WY 82002
(307) 777-7115

U.S. TERRITORIES AND POSSESSIONS

American Samoa
LBJ Tropical Medical Center
Department of Mental Health
  Clinic
Pago Pago, American Samoa
  96799

Guam
Mental Health & Substance
  Abuse Agency
P.O. Box 20999
Guam 96921

Puerto Rico
Department of Addiction
  Control Services
Alcohol and Drug Abuse
  Programs
Avenida Barbosa
P.O. Box 414
Rio Piedras, PR 00928-1474
(809) 763-7575

Trust Territories
Director of Health Services
Office of the High
  Commissioner
Saipan, Trust Territories
  96950

Virgin Islands
Division of Health and
  Substance Abuse
Becastro Building
3rd Street, Sugar Estate
St. Thomas, Virgin Islands
  00802

CANADA

Canadian Centre on
  Substance Abuse
112 Kent Street, Suite 480
Ottawa, Ontario
K1P 5P2
(613) 235-4048

Alberta
Alberta Alcohol and Drug
  Abuse Commission
10909 Jasper Avenue, 6th
  Floor
Edmonton, Alberta
T5J 3M9
(403) 427-2837

British Columbia
Ministry of Labour and
  Consumer Services
Alcohol and Drug Programs
1019 Wharf Street, 5th Floor
Victoria, British Columbia
V8V 1X4
(604) 387-5870

Manitoba
The Alcoholism Foundation of
  Manitoba
1031 Portage Avenue
Winnipeg, Manitoba
R3G 0R8
(204) 944-6226

New Brunswick
Alcoholism and Drug
  Dependency Commission
  of New Brunswick
65 Brunswick Street
P.O. Box 6000
Fredericton, New Brunswick
E3B 5H1
(506) 453-2136

Newfoundland
The Alcohol and Drug
  Dependency Commission
  of Newfoundland and
  Labrador
Suite 105, Prince Charles
  Building
120 Torbay Road, 1st Floor
St. John's, Newfoundland
A1A 2G8
(709) 737-3600

Northwest Territories
Alcohol and Drug Services
Department of Social Services
Government of Northwest
  Territories
Box 1320 - 52nd Street
6th Floor, Precambrian
  Building
Yellowknife, Northwest
  Territories
S1A 2L9
(403) 920-8005

Nova Scotia
Nova Scotia Commission on
  Drug Dependency
6th Floor, Lord Nelson
  Building
5675 Spring Garden Road
Halifax, Nova Scotia
B3J 1H1
(902) 424-4270

Ontario
Addiction Research
  Foundation
33 Russell Street
Toronto, Ontario
M5S 2S1
(416) 595-6000

Prince Edward Island
Addiction Services of Prince
  Edward Island
P.O. Box 37
Eric Found Building
65 McGill Avenue
Charlottetown, Prince Edward
  Island
C1A 7K2
(902) 368-4120

Quebec
Service des Programmes aux Personnes Toxicomanie
Gouvernement du Quebec
Ministere de la Sante et des Services Sociaux
1005 Chemin Ste. Foy
Quebec City, Quebec
G1S 4N4
(418) 643-9887

Saskatchewan
Saskatchewan Alcohol and Drug Abuse Commission
1942 Hamilton Street
Regina, Saskatchewan
S4P 3V7
(306) 787-4085

Yukon
Alcohol and Drug Services

Department of Health and Social Resources
Yukon Territorial Government
6118-6th Avenue
P.O. Box 2703
Whitehorse, Yukon Territory
Y1A 2C6
(403) 667-5777

Richard M. Gilbert, Ph.D., a native of London, has taught experimental psychology at universities in Scotland, Ireland, Canada, Mexico, and the United States. He was for many years associated with the Addiction Research Foundation of Ontario as a researcher and writer on the use and abuse of popular drugs—mostly alcohol, caffeine, and nicotine. He has written some 80 articles for scientific and scholarly journals.

Paul R. Sanberg, Ph.D., is a professor of psychiatry, psychology, neurosurgery, physiology, and biophysics at the University of Cincinnati College of Medicine. Currently, he is also a professor of psychiatry at Brown University and scientific director for Cellular Transplants, Inc., in Providence, Rhode Island.

Professor Sanberg has held research positions at the Australian National University at Canberra, the Johns Hopkins University School of Medicine, and Ohio University. He has written many journal articles and book chapters in the fields of neuroscience and psychopharmacology. He has served on the editorial boards of many scientific journals and is the recipient of numerous awards.

Solomon H. Snyder, M.D., is Distinguished Service Professor of Neuroscience, Pharmacology and Psychiatry at the Johns Hopkins University School of Medicine. He has served as president of the Society for Neuroscience and in 1978 received the Albert Lasker Award in Medical Research. He has authored *Drugs and the Brain, Uses of Marijuana, Madness and the Brain, The Troubled Mind*, and *Biological Aspects of Mental Disorder* and has edited *Perspectives in Neuropharmacology: A Tribute to Julius Axelrod*. Professor Snyder was a research associate with Dr. Axelrod at the National Institutes of Health.

Barry L. Jacobs, Ph.D., is currently a professor in the neuroscience program at Princeton University. Professor Jacobs is the author of *Serotonin Neurotransmission and Behavior* and *Hallucinogens: Neurochemical, Behavioral and Clinical Perspectives*. He has written many journal articles in the field of neuroscience and contributed numerous chapters to books on behavior and brain science. He has been a member of several panels of the National Institute of Mental Health.

Jerome H. Jaffe, M.D., formerly professor of psychiatry at the College of Physicians and Surgeons, Columbia University, is director of the Addiction Research Center of the National Institute on Drug Abuse. Dr. Jaffe is also a psychopharmacologist and has conducted research on a wide range of addictive drugs and developed treatment programs for addicts. He has acted as special consultant to the president on narcotics and dangerous drugs and was the first director of the White House Special Action Office for Drug Abuse Prevention.

Further Reading

General

Berger, Gilda. *Drug Abuse: The Impact on Society*. New York: Watts, 1988. (Gr. 7–12)

Cohen, Susan, and Daniel Cohen. *What You Can Believe About Drugs: An Honest and Unhysterical Guide for Teens*. New York: M. Evans, 1987. (Gr. 7–12)

Musto, David F. *The American Disease: Origins of Narcotic Control*. Rev. ed. New Haven: Yale University Press, 1987.

National Institute on Drug Abuse. *Drug Use, Drinking, and Smoking: National Survey Results from High School, College, and Young Adult Populations, 1975–1988*. Washington, DC: Public Health Service, Department of Health and Human Services, 1989.

O'Brien, Robert, and Sidney Cohen. *Encyclopedia of Drug Abuse*. New York: Facts on File, 1984.

Snyder, Solomon H., M.D. *Drugs and the Brain*. New York: Scientific American Books, 1986.

U.S. Department of Justice. *Drugs of Abuse*. 1989 ed. Washington, DC: Government Printing Office, 1989.

Caffeine

Grobbee, D. E., et al. "Coffee, Caffeine, and Cardiovascular Disease in Men." *New England Journal of Medicine* (October 11, 1990).

Kummer, Corby. "Is Coffee Harmful?" *Atlantic* (July 1990).

"New Caffeine Research Findings." *Nutrition Today* (November–December 1989).

Roden, Claudia. *Coffee*. New York: Penguin Books, 1981.

Schapira, Joel, et al. *The Book of Coffee and Tea*. Rev. ed. New York: St. Martin's Press, 1982.

Glossary

acetaminophen N-acetypara-amino-phenol, or APAP; a potent analgesic and antipyretic chemically similar to aspirin yet without anti-inflammatory action

adenine one of the four purines that make up the genetic code in DNA

adrenaline epinephrine, a hormone produced by the adrenal gland that increases blood pressure and is used in the treatment of asthma

amphetamine a drug that stimulates the nervous system; generally used as a mood elevator, energizer, antidepressant, and appetite depressant

analeptic drug a drug that acts as a stimulant on the central nervous system

analgesic a drug that produces an insensitivity to pain without loss of consciousness

anorexia nervosa a pathological control or denial of appetite due to psychological problems and characterized by excessive weight loss and nutritional deficiencies

antagonistic effect the occurrence of one drug's effects counteracting another drug's effects

antipyretic a drug that reduces fever

apnea cessation of breathing for more than 20 seconds

arrhythmia irregularity of the heartbeat

aspirin acetylsalicylic acid, an analgesic, antipyretic, and anti-inflammatory agent originally derived from plants

barbiturate a drug that causes depression of the central nervous system, generally used to reduce anxiety or to induce euphoria

cacao pods the pods from the tree *Theobroma cacao* which contain seeds used to produce cocoa, chocolate, and cocoa butter

caffeine trimethylxanthine, a central nervous system stimulant found in coffee, tea, kola nuts, cacao pods, maté, yaupon, guarana, and yoco

caffeinism the syndrome associated with excessive caffeine ingestion; characterized by frequent urination, jitteriness, agitation, irritability, muscle twitching, light-headedness, rapid breathing, rapid heartbeat, heart palpitations, upset stomach, diarrhea, and/or heartburn

cardiovascular system the system of the body that includes the heart and blood vessels

central nervous system the body system that includes the brain and spinal cord *cholesterol*   a fatty substance found in body cells and fluids; high levels in the bloodstream are associated with heart attack, hardening of the arteries, poor blood circulation, and a tendency to form blood clots that can lead to stroke

convulsion   an unnatural, violent, and involuntary contraction or series of contractions of the muscles

cytosine   one of the four basic letters of the genetic code in DNA

dimethylxanthine   a xanthine molecule that has two methyl groups; e.g., theobromine and theophylline

DNA   deoxyribonucleic acid, a highly coiled molecule, or helix, composed of two long strands linked by adenine, guanine, cytosine, and thymine, which make up the genetic code

enteral administration   a form of drug ingestion whose route of administration includes the gastrointestinal tract—the mouth, throat, stomach, intestines, and rectum

enzyme   a protein that acts as a catalyst to chemical reactions

epidemiology   a science that deals with the incidence, distribution, and control of disease in a population

fermentation   a chemical process by which yeast consumes sugars, such as those in fruits, and produces effervescence and alcohol

free fatty acids   fat cells that move freely within the blood and can be used for energy by most bodily organs

gastrointestinal tract   the mouth, throat, stomach, intestines, and rectum

gene   sequences of purine triplets within the DNA molecule that code all hereditary traits

glycogen   a complex sugar stored in liver and skeletal muscle cells that is broken down into glucose and used by the body when it requires quick energy

glycosuria   a condition characterized by the presence of glucose in the urine

gout   a hereditary condition characterized by excessive amounts of uric acid (a product of protein breakdown) in the blood which crystallize and are deposited in joints and in kidney tissue

guanine   one of the four purines that make up the genetic code in DNA

guarana seed   a seed from the Brazilian shrub *Paullinia cupana* which is ground to a paste and ingested in a beverage or in wafer bars for its high caffeine content

heroin   a semisynthetic opiate produced by a chemical modification of morphine *hypertension*   a condition characterized by high blood pressure

hyperventilation   excessive depth and rate of respiration leading to abnormal loss of carbon dioxide in the blood

hypokalemia   a deficiency of potassium in the blood

infusion   the steeping or soaking of a substance in order to extract its characteristic chemicals, such as caffeine from a tea leaf

ketonuria   a condition seen in diabetics and characterized by reduced or disturbed carbohydrate metabolism

kola nut   the bitter, caffeine-containing seed of the tree *Cola nitida* which is chewed or used in a beverage

marijuana   the leaves, flowers, buds, and/or branches of the hemp plant *Cannabis sativa* or *Cannabis indica* that contains cannabinoids, a group of intoxicating drugs

maté   a South American holly, *Ilex paraguayensis*, whose caffeine-containing leaves and young shoots are used to make a beverage

metabolism   the chemical changes in the living cell by which energy is provided for the vital processes and activities and by which new material is assimilated to repair cell structures; or, the process that uses enzymes to convert one substance into compounds that can be easily eliminated from the body

methyl group CH_3, a molecule consisting of one carbon atom and three hydrogen atoms, usually found attached to other compounds

morphine   the principal psychoactive ingredient of opium, which produces sleep or a state of stupor; that standard against which all morphinelike drugs are compared

mutagenesis   the occurrence of mutations in a cell, often exhibited as cell character change and/or uncontrolled cell reproduction; caused by mutagens, or mutagenic agents, such as mustard gas and radiation of various wavelengths

opiate   a compound from the milky juice of the poppy plant *Papaver somniferum*, including opium, morphine, codeine, and their derivatives, such as heroin

parenteral administration   a form of drug ingestion whose route of administration bypasses the gastrointestinal tract and instead includes the lungs, skin, ear, or vagina

peristaltic action   successive muscular movements or contractions, such as those in the intestines that move ingested food onward

pharmacology   the study of drugs and their effects on living organisms *physical dependence*   an adaptation of the body to the presence of a drug, such that its absence produces withdrawal symptoms

placebo   a substance that is pharmacologically inactive and is used as a control in experiments measuring the effectiveness of another substance, or is administered in order to satisfy the psychological needs of patients

psychoactive   altering mood and/or behavior

psychological dependence   a condition in which the drug user craves a drug to maintain a sense of well-being and feels discomfort when deprived of it

purine   the parent compound, $C_5H_4N_4$, of such compounds as adenine, guanine, xanthine, and trimethylxanthine, or caffeine

receptor site   specialized areas located on dendrites that, when bound by a specific number of neurotransmitter molecules, produce an electrical charge

REM sleep   rapid-eye-movement sleep; the phase of sleep, characterized by a specific type of electrical activity in the brain, during which dreaming takes place

solvent   a substance that is capable of dissolving one or more other substances; e.g., methylene chloride is a solvent used to extract caffeine from coffee beans

synergism   when two drugs together produce effects greater than either one could produce alone

synaptic gap   the space between the axon and the dendrite of two adjacent neurons in which neurotransmitters travel

tachycardia   rapid heart or pulse rate

tea polyphenol oxidase   an enzyme present in the sap of tea leaves that changes the flavor and color of the leaves, thus producing black tea's characteristic taste and appearance; in green tea this chemical has been destroyed

theobromine   a dimethylxanthine found in cocoa products, tea, and kola nuts whose effect on the body is similar, though only one-tenth as stimulating as caffeine

theophylline   a dimethylxanthine found in small amounts in tea whose stimulatory effect on the heart and breathing is stronger than caffeine; medically used in treating diseases in which breathing is difficult, such as asthma, bronchitis, and emphysema

thymine   one of the four basic letters of the genetic code in the DNA molecule

tolerance   a decrease of susceptibility to the effects of a drug due to its continued administration, resulting in the user's need to increase the drug dosage in order to achieve the effects experienced previously

toxic causing temporary or permanent damage to cells or organ systems of the body

tranquilizer a drug that has calming, relaxing effects

uric acid the main excreted substance produced by the breakdown of protein

Valium an antianxiety tranquilizer

ventricular fibrillation very rapid uncoordinated contractions of the ventricles of the heart resulting in a loss of synchronization of heartbeat and pulse

withdrawal the physiological and psychological effects of discontinued use of a drug

xanthine dioxypurine, $C_5H_4N_4O_2$, a purine that is an intermediate product of the liver's breakdown of the more complex purines to uric acid

yaupon cassina, the plant *Ilex cassine* or *Ilex vomitoria*, whose caffeine-containing leaves and berries are used to make a tea

yoco bark the plant *Paullinia yoco* whose caffeine-containing bark is used to make a tea

Index

0 0 6 4 0 0 2

CAFFEINE THE MOST PO
PULAT STIMULA
GILBERT